Child Protection and Adult Mental Health

For Jonathan and Gavin Wolfe,
Naomi and Eleanor Weir,
and Margaret, Sarah and Gemma Douglas

Child Protection and Adult Mental Health

Conflict of Interest?

Edited by

Amy Weir MA (Oxon) MBA (OBS) CQSW
Children's Services Manager
London Borough of Camden
London
UK

and

Anthony Douglas BA CQSW
Executive Director of Community Services
London Borough of Havering
Romford
Essex
UK

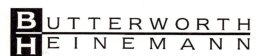

BUTTERWORTH
HEINEMANN

OXFORD   AUCKLAND   BOSTON   JOHANNESBURG   MELBOURNE   NEW DELHI

Butterworth-Heinemann
Linacre House, Jordan Hill, Oxford OX2 8DP
225 Wildwood Avenue, Woburn, MA 01801-2041
A division of Reed Educational and Professional Publishing Ltd

A member of the Reed Elsevier plc group

First published 1999
© Reed Educational and Professional Publishing Ltd 1999

British Library Cataloguing in Publication Data
A catalogue record for this book is available from the British Library

ISBN 0 7506 2904 5

Typeset by Tek-Art, Croydon, Surrey
Printed and bound in Great Britain by Biddles Ltd, Guildford, Surrey

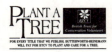

PLANT A TREE
British Trust for Conservation Volunteers
FOR EVERY TITLE THAT WE PUBLISH, BUTTERWORTH-HEINEMANN
WILL PAY FOR BTCV TO PLANT AND CARE FOR A TREE.

Contents

Contributors   vii

Preface   xv

Acknowledgements   xvii

1 An introduction to the issues: a new holistic approach outlined   1
   Amy Weir

2 The real risks children face: the role and perspective of the child psychiatrist 10
   Carole Ann Kaplan

3 Families coping with mental health problems: the role and perspective of
   the general adult psychiatrist   17
   Anne Bird

4 Professional challenges and dilemmas   23
   Elizabeth Parker

5 Parenting as a civil right: supporting service users who choose to have
   children   28
   Liz Sayce

6 Risk assessments of infants born to parents with a mental health problem
   or a learning disability   49
   Lucy A. Henry and R. Channi Kumar

7 Postnatal depression in the context of changing patterns of childcare: the
   implications for primary prevention   63
   John L. Cox

8 Working with parents with mental health problems: management of the
   many risks   69
   Alison Beck-Sander

 9 Understanding the needs of children and families from different cultures   78
    Annie Yin-Har Lau

10 The user's perspective: the experience of being a parent with a mental
    health problem   96
    Nigel Phillips and Richard Hugman

11 The size of the task facing professional agencies   109
    Jennifer Bernard and Anthony Douglas

12 Crossing over between services: the Lewisham experience   137
    Marie Diggins

13 The contribution of the voluntary sector to innovation and development   156
    Christopher P. Hanvey (with an introduction by Amy Weir)

14 Providing services to children and families where the parent has a mental
    health problem: the Australian experience   163
    Vicki Cowling

15 Managing strategies for change in childcare and mental health services in
    Bath and North East Somerset   173
    Maurice Lindsay, Robert G. Potter and Annie Shepperd

16 Building bridges: lessons for the future   182
    Anthony Douglas

Bibliography and further reading   189

Index   205

Contributors

Editors

Amy Weir MA (Oxon), MBA (OBS), CQSW

Amy Weir is Children's Services Manager, London Borough of Camden. Having read history at Somerville College, Oxford, she stayed on in Oxford and began her social work career working in a children's home. She has worked in several different local authorities as a social worker and service manager. She has also managed child health and community nursing services in Islington. Before joining Camden she was Director of Family and Community Care at the Family Welfare Association (FWA).

During her time at FWA, she was involved in organizing two national conferences and in developing services to meet the needs of families affected by mental illness. More recently she has contributed to the evaluation and writing of the Department of Health's new training pack *Crossing Bridges*.

Anthony Douglas BA, CQSW

Anthony Douglas is Executive Director of Community Services for the London Borough of Havering. He studied at Oxford University and the Open University. He worked as an economist and a journalist before becoming a social worker, and then a manager of social services, working in a number of London Boroughs before joining Havering in 1996. He is co-author of *Caring and Coping*, published by Routledge in 1998, about British social services and he is currently writing a similar book on British local government. He is a member of the Association of Directors of Social Services Executive Council and its Children and Families Committee. He is chair of the management committee of the Inner and North London Guardian Ad Litem Panel, and a member of the Council of Counsel and Care.

Contributors

Chapter 2

Carole Ann Kaplan MB, BCHIR, MRCPsych

Dr Carole Kaplan is a Senior Lecturer and Consultant in Child and Adolescent Psychiatry in the Department of Child Health, University of Newcastle-upon-Tyne, and the Fleming Nuffield Unit.

She has a special interest in child protection, childhood depressive disorders, temperament and the treatment of child psychiatric disorders.

In 1993, she was appointed to the Council on Tribunals and has a great interest in the interface between clinical and legal work, an area in which she has given both published and oral presentations.

In 1997, she was appointed to the Lord Chancellor's Advisory Board on Family Law which has the task of monitoring and supervising the implementation of the 1997 Family Law Act and also the Children Act 1989.

Chapter 3

Anne Bird CRCP, MRCS, MBBS, MRCPsych

Dr Anne Bird is a Consultant General Adult Psychiatrist and Honorary Senior Lecturer at the Royal Free Hospital in London. She has a particular interest in training issues and is Organizing Tutor for the Royal Free and Associated Hospitals Training Scheme and Chairman of the Tutor's Sub-Committee at the Royal College of Psychiatrists. From her experience in her clinical work she has set up a Liaison Clinic with the Child and Adolescent Department of Psychiatry at the Royal Free Hospital. She is a member of the Mental Health Act Scoping Study Review Team.

Chapter 4

Elizabeth Parker MB, BCHIR, MRCPsych

Dr Liz Parker is a consultant psychiatrist employed within the Adult Mental Health Directorate of the Lewisham and Guys Mental Health NHS Trust. She is based within a community mental health centre in Lewisham, working with a multidisciplinary team which offers a service to the population of central and east Lewisham. Between 1994 and 1997 she was a Member of the Mental Health Act Commission. She is a senior lecturer in psychiatry at Guy's, King's and St Thomas' Schools of Medicine, Dentistry and Biomedical Sciences. She is currently Programme Director for the UMDS Higher Training Scheme in general and Old Age Psychiatry.

Chapter 5

Liz Sayce BA, MSc, CQSW

Liz Sayce was Policy Director of MIND 1990–1998. She was responsible for policy development, public information services, legal advice and representation, parliamentary liaison, the development of MINDlink (MIND's network of users of mental health services across England and Wales) and Diverse Minds (a new initiative, part-funded by the Department of Health, to improve the quality of mental health services for people from minority ethnic communities). She has a background in social work and mental health policy research and has written and spoken widely on subjects including the development of community mental health centres in the UK, public attitudes and media representations, employment and housing opportunities, and parenting by people with mental health problems.

In 1995/6, she spent one year in the US on a Harkness Fellowship studying the impact of the Americans with Disabilities Act 1990 on people with mental health problems, and other approaches to combating discrimination and stigma.

She is now Health Action Zone director for Lambeth, Southwark and Lewisham Health Authority.

Chapter 6

R. Channi Kumar MD, PhD, FRCPsych

Dr Channi Kumar is Professor of Perinatal Psychiatry at the Institute of Psychiatry, London and Director of the Perinatal Psychiatry Service at the Bethlem Royal and Maudsley Hospitals and King's College Hospital, London. His main research interests include psychosocial and transcultural aspects of postnatal depression and postpartum psychosis; investigations of biological mechanisms underlying severe postnatal mental illnesses and the development of methods of prevention and treatment; and studies of the impact of postnatal mental illness on the psychological development of the young infant.

Lucy A. Henry BSc, D.Phil, D.ClinPsych

Dr Lucy Henry obtained a degree in Psychology from the University of Bristol in 1986. She then carried out research into the development of memory in children, obtaining a PhD in child psychology from Oxford University in 1990. After spending 5 years lecturing in child development at the University of Reading, she went on to obtain a professional qualification as a Clinical Psychologist at the Institute of Psychiatry. She is now a Research Fellow at the Institute specializing in learning disabilities.

Chapter 7

John L. Cox BM, BCh, DM, FRCP(Edinburgh and London), FRCPsych

John Cox is Professor of Psychiatry at the School of Postgraduate Medicine, Keele University and Consultant Psychiatrist, North Staffordshire Hospital. He is a former Senior Lecturer at Edinburgh University and Lecturer at Makerere University, Uganda. He has a long-standing interest in Transcultural and Prenatal Psychiatry. He developed the Edinburgh Postnatal Depression Scale and is Director of the Perinatal Psychiatry Service in North Straffordshire.

Chapter 8

Alison Beck-Sander BA(Hons), ClinPsyD, CPsychol

Dr Alison Beck-Sander is a Chartered Clinical Psychologist who is currently working for Pathfinder Forensic Services in South London. Her work consists of the assessment and treatment of mentally disordered adults who have committed a variety of offences. Her particular research interests include investigations into the psychology of psychosis. She is currently involved in running a number of research projects exploring aspects of psychosis including the prediction of violence, prevention of relapse and coping with mental illness. She has many publications in the field of psychosis and risk assessment.

Chapter 9

Annie Yin-Har Lau MD, FRCP(Can.) MRCPsych

Dr Annie Lau trained in medicine and psychiatry in Canada. She arrived in England in 1978. She worked part-time as a Consultant Psychiatrist for 10 years at Pear Tree House, an assessment centre with a small secure unit run by the London Borough of Waltham Forest. Since 1980, she has been Consultant in Child and Adolescent Psychiatry in King George's Hospital and Loxford Hall (CFCC). From the mid-1980s until 1991 she taught on the Introductory and Part 1 courses at the Institute of Family Therapy. Since 1992, she has been Clinical Director of the Child and Adolescent Mental Health Service, Redbridge Health Care trust.

She continues to be actively involved in contributing to the literature and teaching in transcultural issues in individual and family life, both locally and in national and international forums. She teaches on the Advanced Social Work Course in Family Therapy in Kent, the Introductory Family Therapy course in Birmingham, at the Tavistock Clinic and on the Diploma in Child and Adolescent Psychiatry Course at the Institute of Psychiatry.

She has written on ethnocultural and religious issues and is editing a book on South Asian children. She is a regular reviewer for the *Association of Family Therapy Journal* and the *British Journal of Psychiatry*. She has lectured at international conferences in Zimbabwe, Naples and Barcelona.

Chapter 10

Nigel Phillips BA(Hons), MA

Nigel Phillips has had a varied career in social work and teaching. He has been a lecturer in social work at the Victoria University of Manchester, and is currently a social worker in a Community Mental Health Team in Rochdale. His publications are in the field of parents with mental health problems (with Richard Hugman). He has contributed a chapter on men and mental health to a forthcoming book on men, gender and social work.

Richard Hugman

Dr Richard Hugman was a local authority social worker before becoming a lecturer at Lancaster University. He was Associate Professor of Social Work at Edith Cowan University, Western Australia until 1997 when he moved to Curtin University, Perth, Western Australia. He is also editor of *The Australian Journal of Social Issues*.

Chapter 11

Jennifer Bernard MA, CQSW

Jennifer Bernard has been the Chief Executive of CCETSW (Central Council for Education and Training in Social Work) based in London, since April 1997.

She was formerly Director of Social Services for Newcastle-upon-Tyne; General Manager for Community Care for Birmingham County Council Social Services; and she held posts at Assistant Director level with Kent Social Services. She was responsible for the strategic implementation of the Children Act in Kent and the NHS and Community Care Act in Kent and Birmingham. After qualifying as a social worker in Newcastle, she worked for voluntary organizations in the North of England, including MIND. She has always been interested in learning, development and training, and in the coordination of health and social care. She was the Chair of the newly convened Association of Directors of Social Services Mental Health Strategy Group and is a member of the Ministerial Independent Reference Group on Mental Health.

She holds the CQSW and an MA in Social Policy and Social Research.

She is a Governor of the National Institute of Social Work, a Director of the National Development Team and a trustee of CAIPE (the Centre for Interprofessional Education).

Chapter 12

Marie Diggins MSC Social Work, CQSW, Post Grad. Dip. in Innovation in Mental Health, DipApp. Soc. Science

Marie Diggins is a Senior Social Work Practitioner in Adult Mental Health in the London Borough of Lewisham, where she has worked for 8 years, initially as a generic social worker. Since 1992, she has worked primarily with adults with mental health problems and their families.

She has taken a leading role in Lewisham regarding the 'crossover issues' between adult mental health and child care practice, including carrying out local research, organizing training and conferences, working with the voluntary sector to initiate and develop new resources for these families. She has also developed policies on joint working within and between agencies. In 1995, she received a Community Care Enterprise Award for this work. She is currently a member of the project team working on a Department of Health Training Pack entitled *Building bridges*.

Chapter 13

Christopher P. Hanvey PhD, MSc, MPhil, BA

Dr Chris Hanvey is Director of the John Ellerman Foundation. He has worked in both the statutory and voluntary sector, was Director of the Thomas Coram Foundation, Director of Policy and Information at NCH Action for Children and Assistant Director of Leeds Social Services Department. He has also worked in the Cabinet Office, as an advisor on the voluntary sector and de-regulatory issues. With Terry Philpot, he is joint editor of *Sweet Charity*, published by Routledge in 1997.

Chapter 14

Vicki Cowling BA, BSW, GradDipBehav. Health

Vicki Cowling is a social worker and psychologist and is currently Mental Health Promotion Officer for the Eastern Metropolitan Region of Melbourne, at Maroondah Hospital Child and Adolescent Mental Health Service, Melbourne, Victoria. Her professional career began in government and non-government child and family welfare. For 4 years from April 1993 she worked at The University of Melbourne developing and implementing research and project work relating to the needs of families with dependent children where parents have a mental illness. Vicki regularly conducts and contributes to workshops and training programmes on this topic in Melbourne and country locations. She also speaks at national and local conferences and is editor of *Children of Parents with Mental Illness*, to be published by Acer Press in 1999. She is also currently undertaking a Research Masters project in psychology which examines adoption and permanent care placement issues for children of parents with a mental illness.

Chapter 15

Maurice Lindsay BSc(Hons), Diploma in Professional Management, CQSW

Maurice Lindsay is Group Manager (Children's Services) in Housing and Social Services in Bath and North East Somerset. He has responsibility for the assessment and commissioning of child care services and plays a pivotal role in the development of child protection services and training. He is currently involved in the refocusing of children's services.

Robert G. Potter MB, ChB, MRCPsych

Dr Robert Potter is Consultant in Child and Family Psychiatry and Medical Director of Bath Mental Health Care NHS Trust. His particular interests include the development of a multi-agency child sexual abuse treatment team. He is currently involved in the development of services for children with long-term illness and for children of parents with serious long-term mental health problems.

Annie Shepperd

Annie Shepperd is Director of Housing and Social Services in Bath and North East Somerset. She worked as a teacher and youth worker before qualifying in social work. She has worked in a number of London Authorities and as a guardian *ad litem*. She is a member of the Association of Directors of Social Services, chairing the South West Branch, and she is also a member of the Children and Families Committee.

Preface

Many recent cases where children have died at the hands of one or other parent have revealed underlying parental mental health problems. The most sensational cases have been drawn to national attention through the media.

This book has been written for childcare and mental health professionals. Although there will be some limited reference to the legal framework in the UK, the main thrust of the arguments will relate to professional practice in an international context. Apart from the UK, the book will be of particular interest in Canada and the USA. The editors have recently been in contact with a group of professionals in Australia who are working in a similar field and who have been keen to share information and ideas. South African child protection specialists have also indicated an interest in finding out more about this work. The context of ethnic and cultural diversity will be a common theme within the sections of the book, and one chapter is devoted exclusively to this.

The interface between child protection and mental health is an area of professional practice and legal judgement which has had very little formal attention. We believe this is for two main reasons. First, there has been limited collaboration between the professionals working with children and adults. Second, there has been an historical assumption that mental illness plays only a small part in the causes of child abuse. Strauss, Gelles and Steinmetz (1980) suggested no more than 10 per cent of family violence could be attributed to mental illness. Recent concerns about the definition of mental health problems have suggested the need for a revision of this view to incorporate a wider definition of the nature of mental health problems, particularly depression, which has been a feature of major child death inquiries over recent years. There are many separate texts covering mental health and child protection, but none which focuses on the connections between the two.

We have endeavoured to bring together the concerns of researchers, practitioners and managers about provision for parents with mental health difficulties and for children of all ages.

Broadly speaking, these concerns are as follows:

- When does an adult's mental health pose a conflict of interest within a family?
- When does a parent's mental health pose risks for the safety and well-being of their child?
- How does an adult's parenting capacity become impaired in these circumstances?
- What is a child's capacity to tolerate the changed and often detrimental care which she or he may receive?
- How can those risks be assessed and how can they be managed?
- Who decides when those risks become unacceptable?
- What services need to be available to meet the needs of both adults and children in these circumstances?
- How do professionals working in these circumstances need to be trained and supported?
- What can be done to bridge the gulf between the professionals who are trying to meet the respective needs of children and parents?
- How can the different agencies involved ensure consistent practice and good communication between each other?

We have invited contributions from a wide range of experts who are well qualified to reflect all sides of the debate. Whilst the contributors may start off as child psychiatrists, forensic psychologists, or adult psychiatrists, social workers or policy formers, they emphasize the importance of common themes, we trust without undue repetition. Our aim is that this book should identify and promote ways in which professionals from the respective services can work together more effectively while at the same time each is more able to draw upon the specialist knowledge and experience of the other.

The demands of working with parents with mental health problems are some of the most complex in terms of balancing rights, needs and responsibilities. Failure to ensure that the needs of children are addressed at the same time as the care needs of adults are being assessed, can result in inappropriate and even dangerous situations arising for children. At the same time, staff working with children and families need to understand with precision how a particular parent's mental health problem affects her or his parenting ability, when they are quantifying the impact of adult mental health problems on individual children.

We see no signs of these concerns diminishing. If anything, they will grow as family support developments and community care initiatives develop, with heightened levels of risk in community settings. We hope this book will assist professionals and policy-makers as they grapple with these dilemmas, for which there are no easy answers.

Amy Weir and Anthony Douglas

Acknowledgements

Many colleagues have contributed to the development of this book since it was first planned in 1994. To Terry Philpot, thanks are due for framing the original proposal. Anne Hollows gave invaluable assistance with planning and design. Adrian Falkov supported us with advice and guidance at the key stages. Our contributors stayed with us through thick and thin. Finally, we want to thank our respective families, who tolerated the long hours spent between the initial pipedream and the finished product.

An introduction to the issues: a new holistic approach outlined

Amy Weir

Parental mental illness can have very serious consequences for children and the professionals who seek to protect them, as the following everyday press cutting illustrates:

> 'A baby on an at-risk register was thrown to his death by his mentally ill mother after social services decided she was fit to care for him. Daniel Whayman, aged 16 weeks, died after his mother, Lisa, 33, threw him from the 150 ft Orwell Bridge near Ipswich.'
> (*The Times*, 25 February 1997)

Mental illness affects whole families. There are powerful tensions between the rights of children to be cared for and protected and the needs of parents who themselves are under stress due to their mental ill-health. It is not easy to ensure that a balance is struck between meeting the needs of children and their parents. There may well be a conflict of interest involved.

At the same time, there may also be difficulty in balancing the different perspectives of the professionals and agencies in contact with the family. Some professionals may regard themselves as having a primary responsibility for the children whilst others – particularly in psychiatry – may see themselves as attending to the needs of the ill parent. There may, therefore, be an additional conflict of interest and perspective between the different professionals.

The impact of parental mental illness on children

All professionals working with children and adults where mental illness is a feature need to have a general knowledge of mental illness as well as possessing a framework for understanding child care issues.

Many children live at home with a parent who is mentally ill and develop without experiencing any significant suffering. For example, for many years, I worked with a family with two children whose mother, June, suffered several periods of severe depression culminating in attempted suicide. In the last 10 years June had four hospital admissions but always responded well to treatment. She was well supported by her husband in her care of their two sons, aged 14 and 12 years, who are flourishing.

Other children experience more difficulty with a 'shifting quality of life' resulting from the variable responsiveness of parents, their fluctuating energy levels and the resultant loss of authority which may follow.

There is no doubt that mental illness in parents may represent a risk for their children. Indeed, this has been known for over 25 years. Smith interviewed 214 parents of abused children in the early 1970s, and found much higher rates than average of maternal depression, anxiety and personality disorders amongst these parents (Smith *et al.*, 1973). However, the central question today is the extent to which, in the longer term, a parent's mental health problem so reduces their ability to parent that their children's lives become damaged beyond effective repair. When is this point reached? How can this be effectively assessed and managed? These are the issues which all professionals working in the community need to bear in mind whether they are involved with parents or their children or both.

Factors such as the chronicity and the severity of the mental illness help to determine the impact of the parental illness on the child. Several research studies have found that parents who have discrete episodes of illness and who are able to function well in-between with good relationships with their children, have far less difficulty in caring for their children. When the illness of parents is chronic and persistent, there is no respite for the children and they may be continuously exposed to difficult and damaging parental behaviour. The Woodley Inquiry Report (1995) concerning the stabbing of one service user by another in a mental health day centre in Newham, described how the attacker related his own mental illness to the persistent and chronic nature of his mother's schizophrenia and how, as he became older, he became increasingly responsible for her care to his own neglect and detriment.

If a parent's symptoms include aggression and hostile behaviour, then it has been identified that children are more at risk of both emotional and physical harm (Rutter and Quinton, 1987). Parents who have repeatedly self-harmed, parents who have threatening delusions and hallucinations and parents who include the child in their symptoms – particularly in their delusions – may pose a serious risk to the safety and well-being of their children. Some parents may experience symptoms which interfere with their capacity to relate appropriately to their children and they may behave in a withdrawn or irritable manner. Other parents may experience difficulty in caring for their child's basic needs and safety because of the effects of treatment; some medication, such as some of the major tranquillizers, may make parents drowsy. They may find it impossible to attend to the needs of their children, especially if they are very young and vulnerable.

Parental mental illness may have several stressful consequences for children.

Children may be embarrassed and insecure about their parent's illness and find it difficult to involve themselves fully in school and in other activities with friends. They also tend to have little information about their parent's mental illness, and can be vulnerable to bullying and social isolation as a result of negative remarks made about their parent's behaviour or characteristics.

A 14-year-old described to her social worker how she went to the public library to ask for information on mental illness, pretending she was doing a school project on it because, as she said later on :

'I didn't want them to know my mum and dad were mad, did I?' and 'What do you do when your packed lunch is really peculiar?'

Children may be expected to assume an inappropriate level of responsibility for their parent and may become 'carers' for their own parents.

Another 14-year-old girl described her dilemmas about how to cope with her mother's manic depressive illness:

'The worst part is when you're not sure how ill she is and if you should call the doctor or a friend. Sometimes she just sits and cries. My sister had to do lots of housework when mum was ill. She didn't hate mum but she got a bit mad and felt she was the mum, and mum was the child.'

Children may not develop sufficient skills in terms of their own experience of their parent as a model to be able, in due course, to parent their own children effectively.

Children may not receive sufficient care and stimulation to enable them to achieve their developmental potential because the parent does not respond appropriately and sensitively to their needs.

Children may be abused and suffer significant physical and other harm and perhaps be fatally abused.

Some children seem fine on the surface, until subsequent disclosure reveals they have been suffering neglect and abuse and living in fear for years, all the time wearing a mask.

A range of services have been designed to support and assist families affected by mental illness. Many of these services are directed towards working with mothers who experience perinatal illnesses – both psychotic and depressive illnesses. For example, there are well-developed perinatal services in Nottingham, at the Bethlem Hospital in South London, in Keele and elsewhere. Other services have been developed to support young carers. However, there is no universal national provision which parents and children can expect to receive. In fact, there is evidence of a considerable under-resourcing of the needs of families affected by mental illness.

The Department of Health has recognized these shortfalls and in 1996 funded two pilot projects – a resource centre for families in a south London borough, and an attempt to identify what skills and methods of working are most successful in assisting families. A training pack for professionals *Crossing Bridges*, was launched at the end of 1998. Interest in the European context is growing. The Icarus Project (Implications for Children with Adult Relatives under Stress), managed by the Centre for Comparative Social Work Studies at Brunel University, will from 1998 onwards be researching the interface between mental health and childcare in Denmark, France, Germany, Greece, Ireland, Italy, Luxembourg, Sweden and the UK. In each country, researchers from that country will work with two teams or groups of professionals, one representing the perspective of the community mental health services, the other the perspective of the child welfare and child protection services. Interest in the issues across Europe implies a number of academic and professional staff have arrived at the same place at the same time independently of each other. The Department of Health is also encouraging training courses in the UK which recognize that working with children whose parents have mental health problems is an important programme element. Other links between services are being explored. For instance, work is under way at the University of Sussex to improve assessment processes in child protection cases where parents misuse drugs and alcohol, and the Family Welfare Association is looking at the crossover between parents with mental health problems who also misuse substances.

Service structures and the needs of families and children

During the 1980s, there was an increasing emphasis in the social work profession on the development of specialist skills and knowledge and social work is now predominantly organized around clear and separate types of service user need. The main 'care groups' are older people, physical disability, learning disability, mental health and children and families. Smaller care or service groups include sensory disability and people suffering from HIV and AIDS. Whilst the organization of services into this typology has enabled some services to receive dedicated attention for the first time, the downside is that specialization has led to a reinforcing of boundaries between such areas of work as childcare and mental health just when their true degree of overlap has come to be recognized. The needs of parents with mental health difficulties and their children cut across these conventional professional boundaries. As a result, for the most part, services for parents with mental illness and their children are now extremely fragmented. Services are located on different sites, accessed through different mechanisms, and managed and funded by different agencies. It is against this far from favourable backdrop, that individual professional staff and their agencies need to consider how best to target a good fit between interventions and the needs and strengths of any particular family.

The Department of Health has brought together some key themes in a report produced in 1995. *Messages from Research* identified the need for social workers to respond more sensitively and less reactively to concerns about the welfare of children. An example of this would be a shift of emphasis from investigating whether children are at risk of abuse from the parenting of their mentally ill parents towards a starting-point of considering whether the parents have problems in parenting arising from their mental ill-health. Largely as a result of this research, child protection work is being re-positioned within a more holistic context of children in need. There may be a conflict of interest between the needs of the child and of the parent but an automatic assumption that this is the case is unjustified.

A family support approach is still in its infancy, compared with the head of steam built up by the child protection industry over more than a quarter of a century. A number of studies have asked parents to identify what assistance would enable them to cope with their illness, for themselves and for their children.

Hugman and Phillips in 1991 interviewed 24 parents (Hugman and Phillips, 1993). These parents adopted different strategies to cope with their illness and with caring for their children, some of which relied on the support of family and friends, and some of which depended on the coping capacity of their children. Many of the parents would have liked more support from social workers and other professionals. The parents took their responsibilities very seriously.

'If you've a mental health need, you make sure the children are safe because, you know, you are on your guard all the time, so you make sure your children are safe all the time. Mine have phone numbers all over . . . if I didn't have my phone I'd be stuck really . . . because it's like a safety barrier.'   (Hugman and Phillips, 1993)

Many parents welcomed the support they received whilst others felt very undermined by social workers who tended to concentrate on parental weaknesses rather than on affirming parents as coping. One parent described her feelings as follows:

'Social services as it is now, it's all about child abuse. Why don't they practise what they preach? Because it's a government thing . . . there's a lot of degrading in the name of mental health.'   (Hugman and Phillips, 1993)

Hugman and Phillips concluded that 'In all aspects, the key theme is the wish by parents with mental health problems to have their parenting and their mental health needs acknowledged and responded to in such a way that neither obscures or dominates the other'.

A major research project considering the needs of mentally ill parents and their children in Australia set out to ask 57 parents what support they needed; they identified the following service needs (Cowling; personal communication, 1996):

– Help in explaining their mental illness to their children on a regular basis
– Respite care for their children on a regular basis
– Parent support groups to include reassurance about their parenting when they are unwell
– Supportive and practical in-home care which is consistent and dependable when they are unwell

The needs of young carers including the children of parents with mental health problems have been highlighted by a number of studies. Children have identified their needs in these studies. Children need to know their parents are ill and above all that they are not to blame. Sharing concerns with other children whose parents are ill has been useful and so has the opportunity to talk to an interested adult and to go out to a local project. A study by Alison Elliott in 1992 in Leeds called *Hidden Children* identified the needs of the children and she produced a comprehensive list of recommendations as a result of these interviews. (Elliott, 1992).

She listed the following suggestions for improving the circumstances of children:

- An acknowledgment that children's rights and needs are separate from those of their parents
- A commitment to treat children with respect and not avoid their experience because it is too painful
- Sensitivity on the part of professionals to the stigma and associated fears that surround mental health problems, which children are particularly sensitive to
- Culturally sensitive services which reflect the needs of black and ethnic minority young carers
- Adequate and accessible information about the illness and genetic issues
- Support from an adult outside the statutory and professional services, for example, befriending schemes
- Training for professionals (teachers, GPs, psychiatrists, social workers) on the needs of children in these situations
- Information for professionals about support services for children
- Practical help with domestic tasks, for example, home care
- Specialist counselling and group-work for children

One young carer described her needs more succinctly:

'I don't want people to feel sorry for me. I just need people to listen to me sometimes.'

Family support: effective practice with families

In the opinion of the editors, an enabling model for developing a service to support families is required. Various chapters in this book suggest how such a model might be constructed. It is essential to target support to families. We also need to know which families might benefit from support but also in detail what kind of help is likely to be most beneficial. There have been several attempts to consider which families should be provided with services and which would most benefit. Patricia Crittenden has suggested one useful model. (Crittenden and Clausen, 1993). Levels of family functioning are ranked in an attempt to identify the importance of considering the contributions of parents, children and social contexts to the degree of harm or difficulty experienced by children. The aim is to enable more creative solutions to family problems to be sought and implemented. Families are seen along a continuum of competence in terms of meeting the needs of their children. Five different levels of family functioning are proposed.

Independent and adequate

These families are able to assess and manage their needs through their own resources combined with professional support which family members actively seek and use when needed, i.e. parents attend child health clinics and ask health visitors and GPs about the care of their baby.

Vulnerable to crisis

The family needs in the short term (less than a year) information, advice, support or casework, i.e. a mother who is depressed after being deserted by her partner and left to care for children who are difficult to manage.

Restorable

The family needs so much external support that intervention on many levels over a long period of time e.g. 2–5 years, is required. Intensive casework and a substantial commitment of resources will be needed to preserve the family and to restore it to independence, i.e. father is suffering from schizophrenia, there is marital violence and the children are having problems at school.

Supportable

Family needs are so great relative to family competencies and available intervention that long-term continuous case management and intervention are necessary to enable the parents to rear their children successfully, i.e. children have suffered physical abuse from mother who is depressed and requires hospital admission from time to time.

Intolerable

Essential family needs cannot be met by current services and intervention; children must be placed in more supportive environments, i.e. a mother has assaulted her child causing permanent injury and she has regular psychotic episodes when she is indiscriminately violent.

The overall aim of this model is to encourage professionals to consider how problems can be solved rather than to dwell on the problems themselves. Rutter has recently added his support to this approach of considering how to enhance strengths within families by supporting parents and their children rather than working to reduce adverse circumstances (from a lecture by Rutter, held in 1996).

The degree and severity of parental mental illness varies considerably. There is no simple equation between parental mental health and the outcomes for children; the circumstances of each particular family need to be carefully considered. There is a particular need to consider cultural differences and the over-representation of black people in mental health services (see Chapter 9)

Recommendations for future inter-agency collaboration

Many Area Child Protection Committees in the UK and *ad hoc* groups of staff all over the country are addressing concerns about parents with mental health problems and how best their parenting can be supported. We believe there are five key areas which are important for all professionals and agencies to address locally:

- Services need to be coherently coordinated and integrated within and between each other so that there is effective communication, liaison and consultation between them.
- The needs of children and parents must be considered together. Health visitors, teachers, CPNs, GPs, social workers and nursery workers all need to know how to locate advice and support about how to deal with these issues.
- Service protocols between agencies and between specialist childcare and mental health teams may improve communication between childcare and mental health professionals (see Chapter 11).
- Some families will need long-term strategies of support and a variety of different services to enable parents to care appropriately for their children. The role of a wide range of professionals is crucial. For many of these parents, problems will be inter-generational, with possibly two or three generations where mental illness is recurrent. There will also be a linked and strong interplay with social factors such as social exclusion, a lack of supportive partners and a poor quality of life.
- There is a need for a flexible range of resources in the community to support families, namely family aides, home care, home visiting schemes such as Homestart and Newpin, family resource centres, groups for children and parents and respite care. Services need to be accessible and flexible in their approach.

This is an extremely difficult area of health and social care practice, which is often a balancing act between the interests and needs of children against the background of their parent's illness. Adrian Falkov's study of children killed by their parents found that one in three cases featured a parent with a mental health problem (Falkov, 1996). Falkov drew attention to fragmented service provision and poor communication between professionals. It is also clear from that study and from a more recent one in Lewisham by Marie Diggins (see Chapter 12) that both mental health and child care professionals need to develop the skills and confidence to work across service user group boundaries.

It is in the interest of everyone for us to work in partnership, wherever possible with parents. Positive attempts to support families and to work in partnership with them are, in most situations, likely to succeed. Children whose parents are mentally ill have to cope not only with the illness of their parents but also with a growing realization that they themselves may have an increased likelihood of being affected by a similar illness. There is much still to learn about how children cope in such families but in the meantime we have to learn to juggle the interests of children and the interests of parents. If vulnerable families can be supported to care for their children, then those children will experience far less dislocation and they are more likely to maintain an integrity of identity within their own family.

In supporting families, the role of the individual practitioner often receives insufficient attention. It is often the most important factor in a successsful service. A joint study by the NSPCC and a number of agencies in Brent found that users and carers valued having one consistent worker who was willing and able to coordinate services and who unfailingly responded to telephone messages and cries for help (NSPCC, 1997).

Of course, it will not always be safe to keep children at home. Maya Angelou has put very poignantly the dilemma for those of us who have to intervene in family life:

'How is it possible to convince a child of his own worth after removing him from a family which is said to be unworthy, but with whom he identifies?'

Maya Angelou

The real risks children face: the role and perspective of the child psychiatrist

Carole Ann Kaplan

Introduction

Powerful tensions can exist between the rights of children to be cared for, nurtured and protected by their parents and the needs of parents who themselves are under stress and are also suffering from mental illness. This is a difficult area in which to practise professionally. A delicate balancing exercise has to be undertaken in each case so that the best interests of a child who needs his or her parents are safeguarded.

In this Chapter I have separated out those risks that may arise from factors characteristic of the individual child from those factors which arise within the environment and family in which the child lives. Finally I have attempted to address the real-life situation where both intrinsic and extrinsic factors operate. Many of these can be considered to have cumulative effects which could be advantageous or disadvantageous to the child.

Intrinsic factors within the child

Intrinsic factors could be considered to be those which are constitutionally present in the child and are partly the result of genetic inheritance. Research shows that a child of a parent who suffers from a severe form of mental illness, such as schizophrenia or manic depression, carries an increased risk of developing a mental illness themselves over the course of a lifetime (Weintraub, 1987; Rutter, 1990). These children can therefore be considered to be more vulnerable to the risk of mental illness as a result of intrinsic factors.

Temperament has been described as that characteristic within a child's make up which determines his or her style of behaviour. For example, if we compare two children riding a bicycle, one will ride carefully and steadily, the other will career around knocking into things. This is the same activity, but two very different styles of behaviour. Temperamental factors are of considerable importance in the area of child protection. Thomas and Chess (1977) have described three styles of temperament in children. Firstly, those children who are more adaptable and contented and cope quite easily with changes in their environments and the vicissitudes of care given to them. These children are said to have 'easy' temperaments. There are other children who cry more often, do not fit into a routine and are more difficult to care for. These 'difficult' children can be challenging to care for and when this care is provided by a parent who is not well and is under stress, the combination can result in harm to the child, who can at times be at very high risk. One way to think of this concept is to consider that at best the 'easy child' will provoke positive approaches and responses. However it is also possible that the tendency to protest and cry less may result in the child receiving less stimulation and being ignored. On the other hand the 'difficult child' with a strident demanding cry will not escape attention, but this attention may be of a harsh or punitive nature.

Vulnerability may be conferred on a child as a result of other intrinsic factors such as low birth weight and prematurity. These may be of importance as they may 'reduce the range of arousal within which the infant operates' (Field, 1993) and so the child may be seen as more difficult to care for by his or her parents through being less responsive. Children who are chronically ill or disabled may make greater demands on their parents. Children with long-standing physical and mental disability are found more often than other children in populations of abused children, but the reasons for this have yet to be clearly understood. (Ammerman *et al.*, 1988).

There is another worrying group of children who seem to cope in the midst of striking adversity. These are the ones who seem to be 'managing' in a situation where the quality and quantity of care they receive is very far from what most children would need. The factor of resilience is one which is often quoted in relation to children, but I find reliance on children's resilience to be worrying, and liable to lead to false optimism.

What is the risk?

It is important to consider the nature of the risk or risks that a child may be exposed to. Clearly in an extreme situation there is a danger of a child being badly injured or even killed, and this does occur, with infants being particularly vulnerable. The range of damage includes serious physical abuse, sexual abuse and emotional abuse and neglect. The forms of abuse that produce physical changes are perhaps more easy to deal with, in that a concrete form of evidence is more readily available. An important factor is that many children who have been physically or sexually abused have sustained serious psychological harm which can sometimes be forgotten in the flurry of activity about 'evidence'. Emotional abuse may be difficult to identify, but may produce lasting difficulties. We are all concerned about those children who are in the 'grey area' where either physical signs are non-existent or equivocal, and also those children where concern is primarily about emotional abuse and neglect. The common feature for these children is the vagueness of the injury or harm to the child and the difficulty of explaining this in the concrete operational system of the judicial process where visible harm is easier to prove.

In my experience, it is rare for a child psychiatrist to make a diagnosis of a formal psychiatric illness in the majority of children where protection concerns are raised. It is likely that the children may have forms of distress and behaviour difficulties which may not be sufficient to meet the diagnostic criteria for a psychiatric disorder. These children may be failing to achieve their developmental tasks and a phrase which has been used to describe this is 'failure to reach competency'. Perhaps this is a nebulous concept, but it is one which can have far-reaching consequences for a child's life-long growth and development. The formal psychiatric diagnosis which is often queried in child protection is Post Traumatic Stress Disorder. This includes symptoms of numbness and emotional detachment associated with insomnia and hypervigilance with 'flashbacks' or dreams of the trauma and avoidance or fear of anything that may remind the sufferer of the trauma. There may also be disturbances of mood and behaviour associated with these symptoms. Identification of this disorder is important in children who have experienced abuse, but the actual incidence of the syndrome in such children remains a subject of debate.

Environmental risk factors

A large number of environmental risk factors have been identified by a variety of authors, such as Rutter, Kolvin, Hammen and Sameroff. I have taken the liberty of putting together those factors which seem to me to be of importance cumulatively in the literature. These are included in Table 3.1 below:

Table 3.1 Environmental risk factors

1	Mental illness in one parent, and the contribution of the other parent
2	Marital discord
3	Quality of parent–child interactions
4	Level of stress, life events
5	Maternal anxiety, mood, attitude
6	Reduced family/social support
7	Low social/educational status of parents
8	Large family size
9	Child's self-concept, social competence, academic performance
10	Child's placement in care

The idea of cumulative risk has been described more recently in an important editorial by Browne and Lynch (1995) which deals with the risk factors for fatal child abuse and neglect. Their table is reproduced opposite (Table 3.2).

These factors will not surprise professionals but perhaps the most important feature to arise from the literature is the finding that one factor alone is probably not of great importance to a child if there are compensating features. However, should more than one factor be found, the risk to the child is cumulative so that if there are two or more risk factors in a family where a child's care is cause for concern, the risk to the child is multiply increased compared to that of a child in the normal population. In addition, the literature is helpful in showing us that no specific factor is related to a specific disorder in the child and that the risk may be of a more general nature rather than being associated with a particular psychiatric form of disturbance in the child.

Table 3.2 Risk factors for fatal child abuse and neglect (Browne and Lynch, 1995)

1 Child under five years of age
2 Child suffering from non-organic failure to thrive
3 History of abuse or unexplained injuries to a child in the family
4 Spousal violence or discord in family
5 Care-giver suffers from psychiatric illness or psychological disorder
6 Care-giver excessively uses alcohol or illicit drugs
7 Care-giver under stress and/or poverty (e.g. unemployment or criminal activities in the family)
8 Care-giver young and inexperienced

An interesting feature of this work is the potential for both risk identification and the possibility to provide support and prevention. For example, the importance of mental illness in one parent is that it may pose a risk to a child. However, the contribution of the other parent must be considered and this may be positive or negative. For example if there is a mother who suffers from a mental illness and a father who drinks heavily, behaves in a violent manner and spends a considerable period of time in prison, then the father's behaviour is likely to be an additional risk factor in terms of the care of the child. However, if the contribution of the other parent is to provide support, a good quality of care and protection from the deficiencies in care provided by one parent, this is a positive and protective feature in the child's life. The importance of marital discord, the quality of parent and child interactions and the level of stress and life events are factors which are common in terms of adversity in childhood. Professional agencies can help in a variety of creative ways.

Unacceptable risk is found where there is a risk of significant harm to a child. Clearly some ways in which children are harmed are completely unacceptable and require an emergency response, such as if there is a significant risk to the life or well-being of a child. However, as already said, in the vast majority of cases where a parent has a psychiatric illness, such an acute risk is not the issue. The issue is far more a long-term chronic difficulty where it has taken a long period of time for the child to come to the attention of the various professionals and where the risk to the child has had time to accumulate. I will not deal with the meaning of the word 'significant' other than to point out it is at least 'worthy of note' and that the child must be seen in the context of other comparable children.

Specific disorders

It is very difficult to separate out the effects of specific parental mental disorders. The severity of the parental illness is an important predictor of difficult behaviour in their children but a high level of associated psychosocial disadvantage is also of great importance (Sameroff and Seifer, 1990). These disadvantages may include poverty, overcrowding and inadequate housing, unemployment, marital difficulties and other adversities. It should also be remembered that a psychiatric disorder in an individual person may not occur alone and that there is often another disorder occurring at the same time (Robins and Regier, 1991). In Robins' study, 60 per cent of patients diagnosed as having one disorder had at least two other significant psychiatric disorders during their lifetime. Amongst those with a co-morbidity greater than 90 per cent were antisocial personality disorder and schizophrenia.

Alcoholism and other addictive behaviour in parents is very significant for children. The effects which are exerted prenatally are well known, as, for example, in fetal alcohol syndrome. The effect of exposure to alcohol *in utero* is to affect children's development cognitively and to raise the risk of psychiatric disorders in childhood (Reich *et al.*, 1993; Steinhausen *et al.*, 1993). Interestingly, despite the seriously disruptive effect of alcoholism on children's home life, research indicates that the majority seem to cope well (Werner, 1986). However, it must be remembered that for most parents who abuse alcohol their children will remain outside the professional system and as a result these findings may well be incomplete. Certainly this positive finding from the research, should not, in my view, delay the provision of help and support to these children. The parenting patterns of adults who use narcotic drugs are described as being more disturbed, with parents being more over-protective, thus possibly encouraging dependence in the child, and possibly encouraging narcotic dependence in later life. (Bernardi *et al.*, 1989). An involvement in a 'drug culture' and the significant antisocial activities that may be included are clearly not suitable for a child to have contact with. This and other adverse factors must also be considered from the child's point of view.

Rights

The rights of the child are clearly embodied in recent legislation and of course in European and international conventions. Every child has the right to welfare and to grow and develop appropriately. Each child has the right to love and affection, stimulation and care which provides boundaries and safety. Of equal weight in a wider context is the right of parents to be cared for and not discriminated against when they suffer from a variety of illnesses including mental illness. However, parents are responsible for their children and their ability to exercise that responsibility is what often has to be weighed in the balance. The difficulty here is that most children have a need to be with their parents and to know that their parents are also safe and cared for.

Responsibilities

As I have said, parents at all times carry responsibility for the care of their children. In addition there is a duty on the local authority to safeguard and promote the welfare of children within their area who are in need, and also to promote the upbringing of such children in their families by providing a range and level of services to meet those children's needs. A particularly difficult issue is when no formal diagnosis of active mental illness is made currently in a parent, yet there remains a significant restriction of their ability to provide parental care. The issue of 'scapegoating' a mental health patient may then arise, because of genuine concern about a child.

If the parent believes that they are being blamed and punished for their ill health, not only by the professionals involved, but worse still, by their children, then their self-esteem will fall, their sense of guilt will increase and their ability to provide parental care will reduce further. This stress can be manifested in a variety of ways such as aggression, demoralization and giving up or becoming ill again. It is incumbent on professionals to try to reduce and ameliorate this reactive stress as far as possible.

Other professionals also carry responsibility for the care of children, particularly in health and education. Of particular significance to those practising within the health profession is that if an adult may pose a significant risk to a child, a breach of confidentiality may be needed in order to safeguard the welfare of the child.

Time is an important concept under the Children Act which warns us that we must have due regard to the fact that children grow and develop quickly and that children's timescales are shorter than those of adults. However, there is a view that there are some cases (although by no means all) where time can actually be an ally in terms of helping children. Time can be used constructively to determine whether an adult is going to respond to a significant degree to the treatment that is offered and whether they are going to comply and respond in such a way as to make them able to carry on providing acceptable care for their children. Under these circumstances, following constrained and narrow timescales can sometimes be unhelpful.

We should also notice that an adult who has successfully coped with an illness such as depression, may well have a great deal to offer their child who may be facing a risk of developing similar problems in their own lives.

The way forward

There are many constraints and stresses in relation to families where there is a conflict of interest, and where the members of the family are themselves under a high degree of stress. We are dealing with the problems of fragmentation, the separation of systems, a lack of resources and the problems of an adversarial regime in the child-care legal system. Perhaps we could consider the merits of a model where the child and the parent are perceived as being within a balanced system where the needs of each counterbalance in such a way as to produce, firstly and of paramount importance, acceptable care for a child, and secondly, adequate support for a parent in need of help.

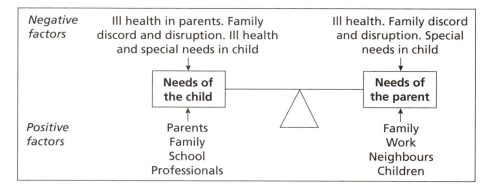

I would suggest that the process of assessment and management must view the child and parent as being within a system, firstly of a family, secondly of an extended family and thirdly, within the constraints of community care. It is my view that if we could identify the supports and stresses in addition to the risks, rights and responsibilities, a way forward can be found to help children and their families in such a way that the child and the parent are both well cared for in an acceptable manner. There will be occasions when it will be necessary to remove a child from the care of their parents who suffer from a mental illness. However, there will be many other cases, where if there are adequate assessment and management planning strategies and sufficient will and resources to meet the needs of children and their families, it will be possible to keep children and their parents together in a way which is mutually supportive and productive, and which above all else meets the needs of the child.

Families coping with mental health problems: the role and perspective of the general adult psychiatrist

Anne Bird

In the final decade of the 20th century there is clear evidence of growing concern within society about the family and the need to identify and protect children from abuse both within the family context as well as those children who have been taken into care. General psychiatrists, have, over recent years, focused their attention on the psychiatric care of the most severely mentally ill following the period of de-institutionalization and development of 'care in the community'. Much media attention has been given to those instances where 'care in the community' has gone badly wrong. Enquiries into these cases and government publications, including *Caring for People* (Department of Health), led to the development of the Care Programme Approach (CPA) to ensure that effective arrangements are made for the continuing care of people being discharged from hospital and being treated in community settings. The essence of CPA is that the needs of each patient, both in terms of psychiatric care and social care, are identified with effective planning arrangements made to meet those identified needs. Perusal of various CPA forms used in different Trusts has shown that there is often no notification made on the forms as to whether the patient is a parent with the responsibility for dependent children. Neither are these issues looked at in the Health of the Nation Outcome Scales (HNOS).

In Britain, as in the United States, women are considerably over-represented amongst those receiving treatment for psychiatric illness. Inpatient over-representation of women is in the diagnostic groupings including depressive psychoses, other psychoses, personality disorders and neurotic illnesses. Analysis of the marital status of psychiatric inpatients shows that married woman are over-represented in this population in comparison to married men.

In this chapter I will discuss the diagnostic groupings of patients which general and adult psychiatrists are involved with and describe the epidemiology and symptomatology of the common psychiatric conditions. This will include the prevalence of such psychiatric illnesses in mothers and a brief discussion of the factors to be considered with respect to the effect on a child of living with a mentally ill parent, although this will be dealt with elsewhere.

'Powerful positive associations to the concept of motherhood typically stand in strong contrast to the negative connotations embedded in the concept of serious mental illness. This opposing valence of emotions and images – caring for others against inability to care for self – is not easily reconciled in a single individual' (White *et al.*, Year unknown.). The question posed by this is, can a mentally ill mother be a good mother?

Prevalence

It has been reported that on the Nottingham Case Register 10 per cent of all new female patients had a child under the age of 1 year, and 25 per cent had a child under the age of 5 years. In our own service in Hampstead, audit of consecutive psychiatric case files showed that 8 per cent of the outpatients had dependent children all of whom were living at home with two parents. Of the inpatient sample 10 per cent had dependent children; 70 per cent of these were in care or adopted, or with grandparents. Of the CPN caseload audit, 16 per cent had dependent children, of whom 25 per cent were on or had been on the Child Protection Register.

Factors to be considered

A number of factors need to be considered when examining the effect of living with a mentally ill parent. These include:

- genetic predisposition
- environmental impact
- exposure to parental psychopathology
- effect of separations/hospitalizations
- physical and/or emotional abuse
- indirect environmental impact
- marital discord/social deprivation relationship (includes relationship with services)
- factors within the child

It is likely that different factors will come into play according to a number of other variables which will include the psychiatric diagnosis of the parent, the parent's level of functioning, the support available to the child and the parent, and factors within the child themselves. There is no clear evidence about the effectiveness of systematic intervention for children of parents with psychiatric disorders.

It has been shown that the psychiatric risk to children is greater when the parental diagnosis is of a personality disorder associated with high levels of exposure to hostile behaviour and emotional abuse. From studies it has been shown that if adverse environmental circumstances improve, children may recover their adaptive functioning, but it may be emphasized that once children develop a marked emotional behavioural disturbance, then these behaviours become less strongly reactive to environmental circumstances.

At present there is little information on and no specific provision made for children of parents with psychiatric illness. For instance, few Adult Psychiatry Departments have close working relationships with Child and Family Departments or with Child and Family Social Work Teams. There is often little provision in adult psychiatry settings specifically for mothers suffering from psychiatric illnesses, although there are of course exceptions in mother and baby units set up specifically to deal with puerperal illnesses.

A general psychiatrist typically deals with patients suffering from the major psychotic illnesses: schizophrenia, bipolar disorder, as well as patients with anxiety disorders, personality disorders, and alcohol and substance misuse.

Schizophrenia is a common condition with a life-time risk of 1 per cent. In Britain a diagnosis of schizophrenia is usually based on clinical features delineated by Kurt Schneider, a German psychiatrist, who identified a number of symptoms which he regarded as of first rank importance in differentiating schizophrenia from other psychotic conditions. These include passivity experiences and thoughts, emotions, impulses, or actions experienced by the patient as under external control. Disturbances of thought control are also included, described as thought insertion, thought withdrawal and thought broadcasting. Auditory hallucinations in the third person is when a voice or voices may be heard discussing thoughts or behaviour (running commentary) or talking in the third person (referring to her or she, or by name), or heard repeating thoughts out loud or anticipating thoughts. Auditory hallucinations are experienced as alien and under the influence of some external force. Primary delusions are part of Schneiderian First Rank symptoms.

Much research has been focused on the aetiology of schizophrenia and it seems likely that there is a genetic basis for genetic and social environmental factors. The risk of developing schizophrenia if both parents are schizophrenic is in the order of 36–46 per cent falling to 13–17 per cent if one parent is schizophrenic. It has been thought that the fertility of people with schizophrenia was lower than that of the general population, however, it has also been suggested that it is rising and may not be different. The so-called negative symptoms (social withdrawal, apathy, lack of social engagement) clearly mitigate against the establishment of close interpersonal relationships. However treatment with the so-called atypical antipsychotics, which came into general use in the 1990s, may alter the clinical presentation and consequent social handicaps of schizophrenic patients. Patients with chronic schizophrenia do not experience the same increase in rate of relapse following childbirth as for instance do bipolar disorder patients (Kendell *et al.*, 1987) Several studies on schizophrenic women and their children have shown that the prognosis in terms of ability to care for a child is generally poor, and aggravated where there is little or no social or emotional support.

In bipolar disorder, characterized by significant symptoms of depression or elation, it has been shown that women who suffer from repeated episodes of mania are likely to have more children than the general population. These women face a substantial risk of relapse following childbirth and pose special difficulties in terms of management in the puerperal period. Estimates as to the prevalence of bipolar disorder vary between 0.5 and 4 per cent. Bipolar disorder is a recurrent illness, with women over-represented with a ratio of 1.3–2:1. Again studies have suggested a strong genetic contribution in the aetiology. Clinically there are episodes of psychotic symptoms, typically grandiose in nature, and elevated mood which may be interspersed with episodes of depression. There is an increased risk of suicide and frequently the need for continual medication with a mood stabilizer such as lithium.

In depressive illnesses, which are the commonest psychiatric conditions presenting both to primary care and to secondary care, the clinical picture is frequently varied but usually has as its hallmark a lowered mood, sleep disturbance, appetite disturbance, poor concentration, social withdrawal and decreased interest and enjoyment. There are conflicting theories as to the mode of inheritance. Genetic factors have been highlighted in cases of moderate and severe depressive illnesses. Again women are over-represented and a national survey of psychiatric disorders in the UK revealed that the prevalence of depression was highest amongst lone parents. Admission rates for women in the age group 20–44 years represents approximately a fifth of all inpatient episodes. The symptom profile of depression has been shown to have an impact on dependent children, 'at the simplest level, the helplessness and hostility which are associated with acute depression interfere with the ability to be a warm and consistent mother' (Weissman and Paykel, 1974). Insecure attachment, developmental delay, educational and social difficulties, as well as the development of specific psychopatho-logical syndrome have all been identified in children of depressed mothers. Sons seem to be particularly at risk in this regard.

Alcohol dependence and drug misuse are common presenting symptoms to general practitioners and secondary psychiatric services. Specific services are frequently commissioned by Health Authorities to manage patients presenting with drug and alcohol dependence but they may also present as a complication of a primary psychiatric disorder such as depression and psychosis. Although men out-number women in the ratio of about 5:1, women seem to be increasingly represented in the diagnosis of alcoholism. Only a small proportion of problem drinkers and drug misusers are known to specialized agencies as parents whose misuse of alcohol or drugs directly affects their ability to care effectively for their children.

Notification of the needs of children of psychiatric patients is imperative. In clinical practice there is acknowledgement that a number of mothers with psychiatric disorders deal effectively and appropriately with their children's needs, both physical and emotional. There are also patients who are unable to cope and they will require assistance. At the extreme end of course, there is concern that illness in the mother may lead to permanent harm or even murder of a child. A confidential enquiry into homicides by the mentally ill showed that 30 per cent of the assailants were female and 40 per cent of those were diagnosed as schizophrenic, and 85 per cent of their victims are their own children (Royal College of Psychiatrists, 1996). However there is no evidence to support the theory that patients suffering from severe mental illness are at greater risk of physically abusing their children than the general population.

Many of our patients have understandable concerns about acknowledging difficulties in the area of parental responsibility. One of their fears is that such an admission will lead to the removal of their children. Whilst this will be an appropriate outcome in a small minority of situations, the overall response would normally be one of supporting the mother both practically and emotionally. This leads naturally to the need for Adult Psychiatry Services to work collaboratively with the Child and Family Services. Both services are stretched, and this works against the development of collaborative work which would be time-consuming and difficult to arrange. There are both training and service implications inherent in these developments, and The Royal College of Psychiatrists have recently decided that experience in Child Psychiatry or Learning Difficulties will be mandatory for trainee psychiatrists undergoing general professional training.

Case studies

Concern involving a particular patient and her child were voiced by neighbours who had heard the child, aged 6 years, crying well into the night and the school were aware of poor attendance, with the child often arriving late and in a dishevelled state at school. Concern had been raised about the mother's mental health and community assessments were taken. The mother, a single parent in her early 30s, had clearly developed a paranoid schizophrenic illness, she was acutely psychotic, experiencing auditory hallucinations, command hallucinations and was fearful of leaving the flat in daylight believing that she would be harmed by a spy under the control of extraterrestrial forces. The child was distraught, confused and anxious about her mother. A formal admission under the Mental Health Act was arranged and the patient had a protracted admission to hospital and proved to have a resistant schizophrenia which responded well to clozapine. The child was cared for by the father who attempted to maintain contact but had been prevented from doing so by the mother's illness. Eventually the child lived permanently with the father and was able to visit the mother regularly following a substantial improvement in her mental state.

Another patient was a young mother in her early 40s with two adolescent children by different fathers. The patient had had a history of eating disorder in adolescence, and in her mid-30s had started to cut her forearms discretely and privately but repeatedly and routinely in an attempt to lose blood and maintain a low haemoglobin which eventually led to a dangerously low level, leading to the patient's admission under Section to hospital. Treatment involved both antidepressants and psychotherapy, and work with the family. The elder son acknowledged that he had had to 'parent the parent'. The family has remained intact with improved contact with the father of the second child who has taken on more parental responsibilities.

A psychologist referred a patient to me who had been seen for a year in the outpatient department for treatment of an obsessional illness. The obsessions involved compelled her to collect rubbish, bits of paper and discarded bags from the street. The psychologist had been concerned that there had been no improvement in these behaviours and indeed the patient had failed to attend a day hospital treatment programme. The patient had three young children, the youngest of which (18 months) had Down's syndrome. They were known to the Child Development Team as there was evidence of failure to thrive. A home visit was undertaken which was revealing. It was difficult to gain access to the house which was on a new estate where the family had recently been re-housed. The hall and each room were jammed full of broken machinery, washing machines, freezers, electrical equipment, piles of rotting rubbish and a cement parking bollard was found in one room. The house was extremely warm and the children all naked. The patient had inveigled her husband, who clearly had mental health problems himself, to bring in the parking bollard which she could not take home herself. The children were all undernourished, and understimulated. Although she expressed warmth towards them, she was quite unable to cater for their needs and the children were subsequently taken into care.

Personality disorder patients form a particular challenge to Adult Psychiatry Services, particularly those suffering from borderline personality disorder characterized by a tendency to repeated self-harm, lability of mood, unstable relationships, fears of abandonment, and ambiguity with respect to sexual identity. A patient, mother of two young children by different fathers, presented with repeated overdoses and self-harming behaviour including cutting of the forearms. In her family background she had been troubled by an absent father, a mother who drank excessively, and a period of sexual abuse from the mother's boyfriend. The elder child in particular was noticed to have considerable psychological problems and was described as temperamental and volatile by the school. Admission to a Family Psychotherapy Unit failed because of the mother's repeated self-harming behaviour and the children were put on the At-Risk Register (emotional abuse). The patient was treated with regular psychotherapy and the children were referred to the local Child and Family Services.

These cases illustrate the types of presentation of mentally ill mothers and underline the necessity to undertake community assessments to identify the health and social care needs of children and their parents.

Professional challenges and dilemmas

Elizabeth Parker

The notion of conflict of interest is very pertinent to professionals who work with patients who suffer from mental illness and who are also parents. For us, the issue centres on where our loyalties lie, and what our authority may be in any given situation. For the adult psychiatrist, it is the adult who is our identified index patient and we inevitably feel that our primary responsibility lies towards our patient and to what we consider to be their best interests.

Exploring the conflicts of interest

Difficulties and conflicts arise when we feel that what our professional judgement suggests is in our patient's best interests conflicts with the best interests or needs of the children for whom they are caring. In an ideal situation, a psychiatrist should be able to address their concerns about the child's welfare with the patient; to talk to him or her about concerns and suggest how to do something constructive to address those needs. In practice, it sometimes happens like this. Patients often welcome the issues being raised, they often have concerns themselves about what is happening and they often recognize the impact of their behaviour on their children. But sometimes, one can find oneself in the difficult and sticky territory of confidentiality and trust. Regrettable though it is, for many people, not just those with mental health problems, the suggestion of having involvement with social services evokes the spectre of their children being removed, with the implied loss of responsibility and control. When we suggest social services might become involved in a constructive and helpful way many patients respond by stating that they do not want involvement; they do not want referral; they are frightened that social services will take their children away.

These are not cases with overt child protection issues. Of course, if we have any concerns about child protection, then we act in accordance with requirements and procedures. The issues described take place when people, who happen to be patients, are having difficulties with some of the practical aspects of parenting. Often what we are suggesting is a contact with social services to provide some extra help with parenting – a place at a nursery or some other kind of help – and very often the reaction or response is a defensive or resistant one which can pose potential problems for our future relationship with patients.

If we make the decision to override their wishes we are potentially harming our future relationship with the patient and with their family. This issue centres upon their perception of the social services. It is an issue which requires recognition both by health and social work professionals. It is certainly not helped by the division and sometimes active dispute between the different elements of social services directorates. In one example of close work with a social worker over a long period, the case was closed by social services following a reorganization. The case involved a woman with a relapsing psychotic condition who had five children. When social services were contacted to re-activate the case, there was a period of about 6 months when the case – and indeed the case file – literally bounced from one office to another as they tried to establish responsibility for this woman and her family.

It is indicative of the situation for those children that they experienced not only the fear and confusion surrounding their mother's mental illness, but also the poverty of their life in terms of practical things – the lack of basic household equipment for example. There was, additionally, the poverty of their experience when her illness led to a lack of basic emotional care. When they were subsequently involved in a research project, one of them remarked that being interviewed for the research was the best thing that had ever happened to her: someone had come to talk to her and spend time with her; they had brought along drawing materials and had taken an interest in what she was saying. That this had been the best thing that had happened to her was a sad reflection on the quality of life for all these children. There was no doubt in this case that the children had not been physically threatened or harmed. It was equally clear that the mother had no wish to neglect them or harm them in any way, but the family circumstances meant that the quality of their life was extremely impoverished and bleak. This was particularly true for the older girls in this family who took on the responsibility of caring both for themselves and their younger siblings.

Commenting on the capacity to parent

One of the questions raised in practice is the question of whether people who suffer from mental illness are capable of being parents. For adult psychiatrists at the sharp end, this will mean providing reports for planning meetings, child protection conferences and courts about whether one of our patients is able to be a parent. There is an irony about this because historically, adult mental health services appear to be designed to discriminate against people who are parents. It is almost as if throughout the system there is a denial that people who have mental health problems can be parents. Traditionally mental healthcare has been provided via inpatient or outpatient services. It is very unusual to find outpatient facilities with a playroom for children. Parents have to take their child into the consulting room, in which case either they feel that they cannot disclose intimate or worrying information before their children – or they choose to disclose this and the children are exposed to inappropriate confidences. Outpatient clinics can be unfriendly places and at times quite frightening. Patients, and those who accompany them, may be sitting in a waiting room and some may behave in ways which will appear strange and may be very frightening to children. If outpatient units are not designed to be friendly to children, then inpatient units certainly are not. Many have active policies that children under a certain age are not permitted on the ward and if they come to visit their parent, the parent may be escorted off the ward to meet them somewhere else.

Overall the theme is that being a parent is not significant and responsibility for considering the issues raised by patients who are parents is frequently denied by the adult mental health services. Some people may be excluded from a potentially useful source of support or help at day centres because they have child-care problems. The same applies to psychotherapy and counselling. Many patients who are involved in regular weekly psychotherapy find that during the school holidays, the therapeutic input is staggered or broken because of a lack of childcare. It is ironic that we are asked to give an expert opinion on parenting when, in reality, it is very uncommon to see our patients with their children. Psychiatrists who visit patients at home will see more of the parent–child relationships but overall the design of the system makes such observations rare, or artificial. It is hard to get an impression of parent–child interaction. Some criticize the adult psychiatrist who either refuses to comment or feels unable to give opinions about childcare. While this may appear to be unhelpful, the issue is complicated.

What can be commented upon

We can make judgements about diagnosis, course of treatment and, with less certainty, about long-term prognosis. It is questionable whether these factors are absolute determinants of whether or not someone may be a good parent. The real issues are dependent on wider issues such as the availability of another caring parent, or the availability and quality of extended family support. Psychiatric diagnosis is not particularly informative in assessing the extent to which positive parenting can be provided. When a psychiatric report questions whether a patient may be able to fulfil the expectations of the parental role, the responsible psychiatrist then has to deal with the repercussions. I am familiar with the experience of writing reports for court which have been perceived as being negative. In one case, my view was that the woman was unable to cope with looking after her children on a day-to-day basis. It took a long time to work out a compromise which allowed us to continue the therapeutic relationship in a positive way. In another case, the patient was expressing concerns about her long-term parenting skills/abilities and my opinion concurred with hers.

There are clearly times when parents decide not to discuss their concerns about their parenting with us in case we breach confidentiality. The problem focuses on trust: on how much information we are entrusted with and on how we are prepared to deal with the confidential information.

Adult psychiatrists and the child protection process

The scenario of child protection procedures and conferences can place a huge stress and pressure on patients' mental health, particularly the uncertainty of waiting for decisions. One of our tasks is to support patients while these proceedings are ongoing. They often feel their needs are not being taken into consideration and certainly are not being given primacy. While the children's needs must be paramount, ideally a balanced approach will enable us to promote the interests and welfare of the adults as well.

Some parents are very sensitive to the effect their illness is having on their children and wish to address those difficulties actively. Others, when their illness is in remission, prefer not to discuss it or to accept that their illness has had a powerful effect on their children. It is hard to know how to deal with the situation where parents can effectively prevent us having access to the children. In some families the children become familiar with the professionals involved in their parent's care and are quite comfortable with us. In others it is quite clear that the parents actively prevent the children from having contact with us. In a study by Dr Adrian Falkov examining children's understanding of their parent's mental illness and the effect of parental mental illness upon the children, the son of one patient, a woman suffering from a recurrent illness, was interviewed. About 6 months later she became ill and had to be readmitted to hospital and, following the usual pattern, the son was sent to relatives, causing disruptions in schooling as well as home life. After his mother had been discharged, and he had returned home, he asked me during a visit if he could see Dr Falkov again because he would like to talk to him. While this little boy was, perhaps, unusual in being able to articulate the need to process his recent experiences, it raises the issue of how, and to whom, children can communicate their feelings. The little boy's mother did not want him to see Dr Falkov, stating 'No, it's alright now, the illness is all over now, we need to get on with our lives.' I challenged this, and suggested that her son was asking to see Dr Falkov because he needed to talk about what had happened. It is a graphic example of how parents who deal with their illness by denying it between episodes, tend to dictate the same way of coping for their children – a cycle which may be difficult to alter or influence.

The ways that illness affects children are multiple and varied. Some patients have a relapsing mood disorder and between these periods of illness they could be well for long periods of time and function very well as a parent. That is not always the case. We set standards for the behaviour of mentally ill parents which perhaps exceed those we apply to parents generally.

Where parents have chronic problems, these both overtly and insidiously affect their children on a daily basis. Perhaps of most concern are those parents who have a chronic psychotic disorder and who involve their children in their delusions. Either the children are part of their delusional system or they expect the children to behave in a way which is compatible with their delusions. So the children are involved in a mad world where reality and unreality become confused and uncertain. More commonly but less obviously there are all the children affected by parents who have chronic neurotic disorders – anxiety states, phobic disorders and obsessional/compulsive disorders. In these situations the way in which the household operates, the family environment, is actually ruled by the parent's disorder. This may not be immediately apparent to outsiders. School refusers may be staying at home to look after mum or dad. Children may be taught that the outside world is scary or threatening or best avoided. These features are not as apparent as a parent who is overtly psychotic. Many people with phobic disorders are accommodated by their families and it will not immediately be realized that the children have major difficulties.

Positive family interventions

Within the health services, our offers of family interventions such as family therapy tend to be restricted to situations where the child is the identified patient. In adult services, we often offer family therapy where there is an adult with psychiatric problems who is still living with ageing parents. But we do not offer it where there is a significantly unwell parent with small children. There is also the question about the impact of parental mental illness and the ways in which it can influence succeeding generations and what children learn or do not learn from the experience of having a parent in a family who is mentally ill.

One patient, a third generation member of a family in which several family members suffer from schizophrenia, describes childhood memories of his mother. She was constantly being admitted to hospital, constantly hallucinating, behaving in a way that was embarrassing and humiliating – going out naked into the street – and in one case he locked himself away because she thought he had stolen his cigarettes and chased him with a carving knife. The family members were ridiculed by other people in the street and for him one of the greatest issues is about being laughed at.

Someone who has an acute psychotic illness may not be allowing their child to leave the house. They may respond to medication and no longer harbour delusional beliefs but they may as a consequence be very sleepy and lethargic. They may not get up in the mornings. If their child has been received into the care system, there will then be a question about whether the child should come home. It is necessary to weigh up a number of issues, including the impact of the separation and how much the mother wants the child home. We will also have to recognize the fact that she may be better in that she is no longer actively psychotic, but she may not be well enough to parent – either through medication or the illness – and that is the point where inter-professional work can identify needs and the ways in which resources can be provided. Twice-weekly CPN visits will not get the child to school, and the family aide will not be able to monitor the use and side-effects of medication. So if the family aide finds the mother stiff and shaky and unable to get out of bed, then she knows who to get hold of. Ultimately the issue is to reduce the distress and dysfunction for both parents and children.

Often people can do well, or well enough, while they are receiving help, but when the input is reduced often there is another crisis. There must be a clear recognition of the long-term nature of the commitment which is required. People suffering from significant mental health problems will benefit from reliable and consistent support, for themselves and for their families, both to alleviate immediate difficulties and as an investment in their children's own future mental health and well-being.

5

Parenting as a civil right: supporting service users who choose to have children

Liz Sayce

Introduction

'Mom was in and out of private and state psychiatric hospitals until I was about eighteen years old. But in spite of all the trauma, she was able to raise wonderful successful children.' (David Leiker, on the opening of a building commemorating his mother's life, Austin, Texas, 1996)

'The Mothers' Project has helped me enormously – with my divorce, in getting custody of Marlene, and giving me support. You know if you have trouble with your child screaming on the bus you can come here and talk about it and people will say, they've been through that too. And you learn more about how to be a good parent. I've seen a lot of people get custody of their children, or get unsupervised visits.' (User of the Thresholds Mothers' Project – a project that supports people with mental health problems and their children – Chicago, 1996)

Beginning a discussion of parenting by people with mental health difficulties with 'successes' goes against the grain of our culture's prejudices. These quotes voice experiences that are usually totally unheard of. In the media, in ordinary conversation, and even in professional literature, we almost never hear about the people with mental health problems who bring up children well, or well enough; nor about those who can do so providing they have support. This is because there is an entrenched cultural belief that people diagnosed mentally ill should not reproduce and cannot parent.

It is the contention of this chapter that at this point in history we need to break that assumption. We may now have begun to recognize that people with mental health problems are citizens who can live in ordinary housing, undertake work and exercise the right to vote. But parenting by people with mental illness, as well as parenting by people with a severe learning disability, remains one of the last taboos: citizenship stops short of the opportunity to reproduce and raise children.

This chapter proposes a framework for extending citizenship rights to the field of parenting, based on principles of anti-discrimination and access to opportunities to parent. This model can be used to address the rights of parents and potential parents in conjunction with the best interests of children and the interests of the wider society.

It is time to put an end to experiences like the following – described by Kay Jamison, professor of psychiatry and mental health service user:

> 'In an icy and imperious voice that I can hear to this day, he (the physician) stated – as though it were God's truth, which he no doubt felt that it was – "You shouldn't have children. You have a manic-depressive illness". I felt sick, unbelievably and utterly sick, and deeply humiliated. Determined to resist being provoked into what would, without question, be interpreted as irrational behaviour, I asked him if his concerns about my having children stemmed from the fact that, because of my illness, he thought I would be an inadequate mother or simply that he thought it was best to avoid bringing another manic-depressive into the world. Ignoring or missing my sarcasm, he replied "Both". I asked him to leave the room, put on the rest of my clothes, knocked on his office door, told him to go to hell, and left. I walked across the street to my car, sat down, shaking, and sobbed until I was exhausted.'
>
> (Jamison, 1995)

Physicians and others in positions of power over service users need to know that experiences like David Leiker's, quoted above, are a possibility. Otherwise they will continue to make decisions based on spurious generalizations. They need to know that being diagnosed with manic depression, schizophrenia or another mental disorder does not have to be a bar to having and bringing up children.

Unfortunately, to date, we have not thrown off the legacy of the prohibition on childbearing by people with mental health problems, which has stretched across much of the 20th century.

Worthy and unworthy lives

A few decades ago, people who were 'insane, idiotic, imbecile, feeble-minded or epileptic' were forcibly stopped from breeding through compulsory sterilization programmes. In the US, from 1907 onwards, approximately 60 000 people – women, men and children – were forcibly sterilized, often without being informed of what was being done to them (Lombardo, 1983). Gould documents how one woman, Doris, was told that her operation was for appendicitis. In 1980 she learnt otherwise and was now 'with fierce dignity, dejected and bitter because she had wanted a child more than anything else in her life and had finally, in her old age, learned why she had never conceived' (Gould, 1985).

The long-term aim of the sterilization programmes was to rid society of the burden of people who were 'inadequate'. Hereditary mental defects were thought to be linked to assorted social ills such as crime, prostitution and drunkenness (Lombardo, 1985).

A landmark Supreme Court case in 1927 upheld the right forcibly to sterilize Carrie Buck who was purportedly 'feeble-minded'. Judge Holmes, reflecting in his judgment that our 'best' citizens may be called on to give up their lives in war, said of sterilizing the feeble-minded or insane:

> 'It would be strange if we could not call upon those who already sap the strength of the state for these lesser sacrifices...It is better for all the world, if instead of waiting to execute degenerate offspring for crime, or to let them starve for their imbecility, society can prevent those who are manifestly unfit from continuing their kind . . . Three generations of imbeciles are enough.'   (Gould, 1985)

A secondary aim was to free some of those currently locked in institutions, to save money and to enable them to work. Lombardo quotes Virginia General Hospital Board notes from 1923 stating that an aim of sterilization was 'to relieve the institutions of their crowded conditions (and in order that inpatients) could leave the institutions, become producers and not propagate their kind' (Lombardo, 1985).

Of course, sterilization was only necessary to their release if one assumed they should not 'propagate'. Underlying all the arguments was the presumption that it is socially desirable to prevent the creation of new human beings who might be mentally ill or feeble-minded. They might diminish the gene pool, they might contribute to crime and prostitution, and they might be expensive.

Critics of the sterilization programmes have noted that they were used to control reproduction by poor whites and by African Americans. For instance, Lombardo has shown that Carrie Buck was of average intelligence. She was targeted because she was poor and pregnant – by rape, a fact entirely overlooked by the court as they deliberated on her promiscuity and carelessness. Her mother and daughter were also not 'imbeciles' as claimed. Her lawyer and the hospital that ordered the sterilization were in collusion; the entire trial was a charade (Lombardo, 1985).

There is a risk with this type of argument: it can be used to imply that it was more acceptable to sterilize someone who really was 'insane' or 'feeble-minded' than someone who was simply black or poor. In an otherwise illuminating television documentary on Virginia's sterilization programme broadcast in the early 1990s, a spokesperson for the American Civil Liberties Union stated that if sterilizing people with disabilities was wrong, it was even worse to sterilize people who were not disabled. This suggests that even in the current era, a television programme showing the shocking fact that people who were not disabled were sterilized may be more marketable than a programme showing that people who were disabled suffered this abuse.

In Britain there was no mass sterilization programme but there was considerable support for the idea – from, amongst others, George Bernard Shaw, the Webbs and Winston Churchill.

In Nazi Germany in the 1930s, policy makers adapted Virginia's laws with enthusiasm. At least 350 000 people, categorized most commonly as feeble-minded, schizophrenic or epileptic, were sterilized in Germany in the 1930s (United States Holocaust Memorial Museum, 1996). Estimates of the total number sterilized in

Europe during the Nazi era are uncertain; some put the figure as high as 2 million (Blum, 1995).

Dr De Jarnette, who had been instrumental in introducing the law in Virginia, looked to the German example and pressed for increased use of the Virginian law, noting that: 'No person unable to support himself on account of his inherited condition has a right to be born' (Lombardo, 1983).

In Germany it was a logical next step – and one that could be introduced without too much opposition as war approached – to start mass killing of existing children and adults with disabilities. This was euphemistically called the euthanasia programme. People considered 'useless eaters' and 'life unworthy of life' were gassed in ex-psychiatric hospitals, or killed by lethal injection, or shot. At least 250 000 people with mental or physical disabilities were killed in these programmes from 1939 onwards, in Germany and its occupied territories. Records from the era show meticulous calculation of the savings in potatoes, margarine, quark and jam from those people who had been 'disinfected' (killed). School mathematics books posed questions including: 'the construction of a lunatic asylum costs 6 million marks. How many houses at 15 000 marks each could have been built for that amount?' The lives of people with problems like schizophrenia and manic depression had been declared not worth the expense (United States Holocaust Memorial Museum, 1996).

The fact that staff at Hadamar celebrated the cremation of their 10 000th inpatient in 1941 with beer and wine, served in the crematorium, perhaps testifies to the fact that it really had become socially acceptable to rid society of lives seen as a taint on the race and an expense to the State. Terms like euthanasia and 'mercy killing' provided a veneer of legitimization that may have helped nursing and medical staff to accept their role. Photographs of staff from the era – including individual portraits of doctors and a group photograph of nurses at one of the killing centres – give a general appearance of business as usual (United States Holocaust Memorial Museum Resource Library).

Forced sterilization and mass killing are ethically different. It is more grave for the State to commit murder than to restrict individual autonomy in relation to invasive medical intervention and fertility. Yet the philosophical underpinnings in terms of social vision are identical. Both rely on a distinction between worthy life and 'life unworthy of life'. Both justify reducing or eliminating the 'unworthy' for the sake of the economic and genetic 'good' of 'society'.

Bad nature or bad nurture?

One might hope and assume that this appalling history is over. In fact we are still living in the shadow of its ideas.

The Virginia law allowing forced sterilization was repealed in 1974. But just as people diagnosed mentally ill were to some extent freed from the idea that their genes meant they should not breed, they were confronted by the view that they could not make good enough parents. In the 1960s and 1970s laws emerged across the US that curtailed the parental rights of people with mental illness: by 1985, 23 States had laws permitting termination of parental rights solely because the parent was 'insane', an 'idiot' or similar generalized categories (Stefan, 1989). Childbearing by people with mental illness no longer simply spelt bad nature; it spelt bad nurture. However good a parent the person might be, parental rights could be terminated with impunity.

Parents who have lost custody of their children in recent years because of their mental health problems have talked of it as a 'personal holocaust' (Cogan, 1993), a 'kind of grieving like you can only grieve for death' (Jesse, personal communication, Washington DC, 1996). In some cases they have committed suicide as a result (Perkins, 1992). In others the pain has remained with them for years or decades. Jesse, who lives in Washington DC, last saw his son in 1974 and still worries about him every time he hears of an accident happening to a African American man of his son's age – although he does not know if his son is alive or dead. Research in the US and consultation in the UK through MIND's Stress on Women campaign testifies to the awful loss and inadequacy many parents are left with after losing custody, or even after relinquishing children voluntarily. For instance, 'Jill' was not allowed to leave the hospital for the final court case to grant custody to her ex-husband. Her son was brought to her to say goodbye:

> 'They brought him to the hospital and it was just horrible. I cried and cried and cried . . . it was just horrible.'
> (Cogan, 1993)

> 'After maybe a lifetime of coping with abuse and managing to be a mother you are repaid not with care and support when you break down, but by a lifetime of despair and guilt that you have lost your children and let them down. Often there is not even a chance to give an adequate explanation (if there can be one!) as to why "mummy can't be with you at home any more". How these words hurt just to write them and remember.'
> (letter to MIND, Anon., 1992)

In 1996 MIND undertook a survey of 778 service users; of those with children, 48 per cent of women, and 26 per cent of men, believed their parenting ability had been unfairly questioned (Reed and Baker, 1996).

We might accept such pain as a social necessity if we were sure that the thinking behind public policies, and the ways in which they are implemented, were free of prejudice and discrimination. We can have no such assurances. But before examining the more recent history we need to have an idea of what policy and practice based on anti-discrimination and access principles would mean.

A new framework

In spheres of life other than parenting – for instance, employment – anti-discrimination and access principles have been articulated, debated, to some extent codified in law and to some extent implemented. In parenting this process has hardly begun. Some of the principles are, however, transferable.

In employment, anti-discrimination principles mean that if a disabled person can do a job – if they are 'qualified' – they should have the opportunity to do so without discrimination. They may need an 'accommodation' to make it possible – like changing a rota for someone whose medication makes them unable to work an early shift. They may also need to be in supported employment – for instance, having support inside or outside the workplace to help them deal with structuring their work, dealing with the workplace culture and so forth. By analogy, a person who is potentially able to parent well enough (according to the legal standards expected of everyone else) – should not face discrimination. She or he may need accommodations, like respite child care during episodes of severe depression. He or she may also need to be supported in order to parent: by having help in the home, or outside it – as happens, for instance, in the intensive programmes available at the Thresholds Mothers' Project in Chicago.

Principles of anti-discrimination are enshrined in law in both the US (the Americans with Disabilities Act, 1990) and the UK (the Disability Discrimination Act, 1995). Both cover psychiatric disability. Neither requires the type of intensive supported employment or supported parenting described above, but they do require accommodations – for instance, the ADA requires employers to make accommodations, providing they do not cause 'undue hardship' to the employer (Rubenstein, 1993; Gooding, 1995).

Working according to anti-discrimination principles does not mean neglecting the interests of the child. A parent has to be able to parent – perhaps with a lot of support – just as an employee has to be able to do a job. What anti-discrimination principles do mean is that parents who are disabled should never be expected to meet higher standards of parenting than anyone else. And access principles mean they should be supported in order to have the opportunity to parent.

Some might wish to argue that, in any conflict between the interests of the child and the rights of the parent, the child's interests should prevail. There are several problems with this. First, the conflict is often not just between these two parties. For instance, in Chicago a specialist interdisciplinary team assesses risk in cases of parental mental health problems. If the mother, or father, has no support network, no housing that accepts a baby, no access to childcare, no respite childcare available when she needs to go into hospital – then the child may have to be fostered, perhaps for years. If, however, we as a society funded those services – and in many places we do not – then her interests and those of the child might coincide.

A mental health consumer from Texas told me that she spent years being afraid that her three children would be taken away; and the children were afraid 'that the men in the ambulance might come for her again and they would not know whether they would see her again'. She had been offered no help with her children.

Of course there can also be real conflicts of interest: but they are not all simply between a parent and a child. Perkins describes how Anita, a woman with severe mental health problems, had her child adopted. She was then allowed no contact with the child, supposedly in the child's interests (Perkins, 1992). Total severance is only occasionally in a child's interests. It may more often be in the interests of the adoptive parents: so here we have another third party in the complex interplay of interests.

We need a model for decision-making that openly acknowledges the complexity of all these interests and does not reduce everything to an over-simplified conflict between child and parent. It is also an over-simplification to concentrate on the interests of the child to the exclusion of others. Stefan (1989) has shown that the concept of the 'best interests of the child' is so broad that judges can easily slip all kinds of prejudicial attitudes into its definition. A judge may well assume, for instance, that it is not in the best interests of the child to be brought up by a parent with schizophrenia. This can only be corrected for by ensuring that anti-discrimination principles are adhered to in decision-making: they are not secondary to a (potentially discriminatory) definition of the best interests of the child.

It may be objected that people with psychiatric impairments really do have problems in being parents: they may transmit their impairment genetically; and they may be unable some or all of the time to parent adequately. On this argument, to recognize these facts is not to be discriminatory, but to reflect the reality of disability. But there is no evidence that suggests that these problems are of a nature or degree to warrant generalized conclusions about whether people with mental health problems can or should parent.

Assumptions and evidence

Evidence on genetic predisposition to psychiatric disability is not conclusive, but even those most convinced by the methodologies of studies so far suggest that if, say, a person diagnosed schizophrenic has a child, that child may have as high as a 10 per cent chance of developing schizophrenia (McGuffin *et al.*, 1995). In other words, they may have a 90 per cent chance of not developing it. Even if they do, does that mean they should not be born? As the disability community has so eloquently put it, it is not necessarily better to be dead than disabled (Golden, 1991).

If we look at evidence on childrearing by people diagnosed mentally ill, we find incomplete information. Mowbray *et al.* (1995), in reviewing research on mothers with mental health problems, notes some specific parenting problems, but equally some under-researched examples of women raising children successfully; and evidence of a lack of economic and social resources for the women concerned. Most studies do not control for poverty and other social stressors, which Oyersman *et al.* found to be a better predictor of child development than any mental illness measure (Oyersman *et al.*, 1992). Doleman (1987) found a group of children of parents with severe mental illness who not only thrived but excelled, sometimes through finding other adult support in addition to that of their parents. Mowbray also found a startling neglect by mental health services of these women's needs. One survey of State mental health departments found that less than a third even recorded the existence of the children of their service users (Nicholson *et al.*, 1993). MIND similarly found that in one health region in England most social services records for adults with mental health problems had no space to record children or other dependants. There was a category for carers. People with mental health problems, in the old paternalistic tradition, are assumed to be dependent, not to have dependants (Sayce, 1996).

Available research does not ascertain the quality of parenting by people with mental health problems who do have support. This is because support is so often not forthcoming, and has been little studied. With the exception of a handful of projects like the Chicago Mothers' Project, there is little effort, equivalent to the rehabilitation effort to help people find and keep jobs, to support people to have and raise children. In the UK, greater efforts are made, sometimes under court direction, to offer family support packages, including the use of placements in residential family assessment centres as a last ditch attempt to keep families together when they are on the brink of collapse.

Research on the contribution of psychiatric problems to violence – committed against anyone – shows that mental health problems are far less significant than use of alcohol or illegal drugs, being young and male, or poverty (Sayce, 1995). Work on the contribution of psychiatric disability to violence against children in particular is not conclusive. It has not fully separated out the impact of drug and alcohol use, poverty and other social stressors, and psychiatric problems *per se*. Falkov concludes his review on this subject by urging further research, more support for parents and children at risk and improved inter-agency collaboration. He notes a range of parenting abilities, including impressive coping despite significant adversity.

Discrimination in practice

At present the anti-discrimination and access model is a pipedream. Apparent moves have been made, but they amount to little.

Since the 1980s some State laws defining mental illness *per se* as sufficient grounds for terminating parental rights have been struck out. In addition, the introduction of the Americans with Disabilities Act 1990 should protect people with disabilities, including psychiatric disabilities, from discriminatory decisions on the part of public bodies. In practice people continue to lose custody of their children as they did before. Stefan (1989) shows that parents diagnosed mentally ill lose custody 'under fact situations that would rarely constitute grounds for termination with "normal" parents, such as bad attitude or sexual promiscuity'. She attributes this to pervasive social prejudice against people diagnosed mentally ill, which is shared not only by judges but also by many mental health professionals giving evidence in court.

In the UK MIND reports on one case in which a man with a record of grievous bodily harm – he had broken his wife's spine – was granted custody of a child in preference to his wife who had a mental health problem and was involved in a lesbian relationship. The judge commented that in the back of his mind was the thought that 'if she had been normal' the outcome might have been different (Sayce, 1996). UK research data shows that childcare social work staff are most likely to be cautious in decisions about returning children to their parent when psychiatric problems are involved. Their caution stems in part from a frequent lack of training in mental health (Sayce, 1996). Meanwhile adult mental health staff often know little about the possibilities of setting up extended networks of support and may recommend separation in the absence of sufficient knowledge of best practice in childcare.

Judges and magistrates, also not generally trained in mental health issues, share the fears and tend to accept professional recommendations whether flawed or not. Parents from black communities are especially likely both to be diagnosed mentally ill, and to lose involvement with their children (Sayce, 1996).

In the US Mowbray*et al.* (1995) found that of 22 cases of parental rights terminations that had gone to appeal, the terminations were affirmed in 19 of the cases.

Since the introduction of the Americans with Disabilities Act 1990, legal challenges to parental rights terminations have been universally unsuccessful – often because law on parental rights terminations is seen as more relevant than anti-discrimination law (for instance, State of Wisconsin versus Raymond C 1994). Decisions are made in the 'best interests of the child' – which can be interpreted in a way that discriminates on mental health grounds. Cogan reports that while mothers with mental health problems have to do everything right to be considered adequate, 'every iota of care by the (non-mentally ill) father is overvalued'. Judges may consider care by men to be extraordinary *per se*, and also are inclined to undervalue care given by someone diagnosed mentally ill (Cogan, 1993).

Caplan cites a letter from a lawyer, representing a mother with mental health problems, to a psychologist. He asks whether she is suffering from personality disorder or dissociative disorder as 'obviously the diagnosis and prognosis for recovery would have serious implications for her ability to care for her children in future' (Caplan, 1995). If even the lawyer acting for the woman believes parenting ability can be deduced from diagnosis, the chances of justice seem slim.

Parents with mental health problems themselves speak eloquently about how they feel more 'on trial' about their parenting abilities than other parents; and how this taints their contact with services with layers of mistrust. For instance: 'I knew that if I was not careful how I walked into a psychiatric ward that I may not see my son or the light of day for a long time.' When asked how she knew this, the reply was 'common sense' (Cogan, 1993).

Service providers do not always understand the impact of these fears. Nicholson *et al.* (1996) cite a case in which a woman's feelings that people were after her children were labelled as paranoia in her hospital charts. In fact she was being watched by social services staff assessing her parenting skills.

Caplan reports on several cases of women around the US who decided to stay with abusive husbands – after the husbands had threatened to seek custody by claiming the women suffered from pre-menstrual syndrome (Caplan, 1995). If a woman has or can be made out to have a psychiatric disability, she knows all too well that she may lose her children. As one woman put it to me:

'My worst fear was of losing my children. I think it actually prolonged the mental illness, because I was so scared and there was no one to help with the kids. If only there had been someone there to help.'   (Peggy, Austin, Texas, 1996)

For some women the fear of losing children stops them seeking help at all. This problem is recognized by clinicians and advocacy groups, but little researched. One US study did find it was a major barrier to seeking mental health treatment amongst low income women. One said 'if you've had a breakdown it will follow you faster and further than a prison record' (Belle, 1982, quoted in Stefan, 1989).

A further major problem is the lack of support offered to women, and men, who have children. In part this is because rehabilitation has classically focused more on employment outside the home – especially for men – than on women's work, whether paid work or parenting. As one mother, who had been through many years of mental health inpatient and outpatient services, put it: 'you're lucky if you get a couple of classes in parenting' (Peggy, Austin, Texas). Dr Laura Miller of the University of Illinois has proposed to the American Psychiatric Association that they formally include parenting within vocational rehabilitation, along with other types of work, in their *Treatment Guidelines for Schizophrenia*. So far this proposal is absent in British mental health policy.

It is to be hoped that legal challenges to the discrimination faced by parents with mental health problems will be continued, as the Disability Compliance Bulletin (1996) suggests that they can be under the ADA, and that similar legal developments will follow in the UK.

Until then, we are carrying on the tradition of belief that people who are 'insane' or 'feeble-minded' have no right to raise children. Whilst other individuals do have that right, this group is denied it because it is expensive to provide sufficient support, because their 'nurture' is assumed inadequate (just as their 'nature' was in the 1930s), because their rights can be so easily overruled. Moreover, there is a resurgence of the view that their nature, too, may disqualify them from parenthood.

The resurgence of genetic explanations

Gostin (1993) discusses the case of a Health Maintenance Organization which considered refusing health coverage to a couple if they went ahead with a pregnancy when they knew there was a risk of cystic fibrosis. We are approaching an era in which genetic testing will be a matter of a simple blood test at a cost of $10. As we become divided, as the US Congress put it, into those with pluperfect and those with imperfect genes, there is a major risk that the 'imperfect' among us will hit against walls of policy disincentives to reproducing. Insurance companies may not be prepared to pay. In the UK, where it is generally the state that picks up the tab for health care, MIND (National Association for Mental Health) has already heard examples of genetic 'counselling' by NHS staff being used to dissuade people with mental health problems from having children, rather than to enable them to make an informed choice.

There is no reason to imagine that these problems will be readily resolved. Whilst academic debate over the ethics of the human genome project rages, policy initiatives charge ahead. In the mid-1990s States including Virginia and New Jersey have policies that limit benefits to mothers who have a further baby whilst on welfare – effectively discouraging the poor from breeding. Richard Lynn's view that social programmes to reduce poverty fail because the underclass is genetically handicapped provides a neat justification for reducing social expenditure (*The Independent*, 1995). And as conservative commentators seek genetic explanations for everything from rape to robbery, we may predict increasing attempts to reduce undesirable or 'unworthy' genes from the future population, not only – benignly – to reduce the suffering of illness but also to reduce disability and difference. People diagnosed mentally ill could be caught up in this wider trend. They may be discouraged from breeding for the sake of the gene pool and the economic good of society – exactly as in the US in the 1920s. Mental disorder is already conflated with violence in the media and public imagination (Sayce, 1995). The push to reduce bad genes is likely to involve public debates which treat crime and mental disorder as one – again, exactly as in the attempts to reduce crime and prostitution along with insanity earlier in the century.

Concerns such as these have led some in the disability community to flirt with the Right to Life movement in the US (Golden, 1991), just as some gay people have begun to express anxieties about abortion when people may want to abort a foetus carrying the so-called 'gay gene'. But in general the abortion debate remains rooted in the idea of a conflict between the individual choice of the mother and the right to life of the foetus. This ignores debates about the values of the wider society: for instance, will we fund services for disabled people whose births could have been prevented? Will mothers who do not opt for termination – and their disabled children – be stigmatized? As long as we maintain a simplistic abortion debate focusing on a conflict between a woman and a foetus we do not even begin to grapple with these questions of social value and ethics.

This abortion debate echoes debate on the conflict between a parent and a child in parental termination cases. There is an urgent need to broaden both discussions, in order to sever our link to the history of the eugenic movement.

Meanwhile, people with mental health problems are now being confronted with the view that both their nurture, and once again their nature, disqualify them from reproducing. By the time that Dr Kay Jamison – quoted in the introduction – visited her physician, she was met with the view that both factors made her an unacceptable parent. People with less social privileges than she are even more likely to be discouraged or prevented from childrearing: for instance, because they do not have the childcare and social resources to demonstrate they can parent; or because their housing is inadequate and riddled with cockroaches, as in one case cited by Sackett (1991).

In the 1990s the discouragement of childrearing is subtler than in the 1920s. But it permeates every stage of reproductive and parenting decisions. The following examples show both how this happens and how an anti-discrimination and access framework could work to change it.

Having sex

When people were routinely institutionalized for decades, they were expected to be celibate. Everyone knew they were not and oral histories abound with examples of how in fact people had sex in the hospital grounds, bartered sex for cigarettes and so forth. 'Promiscuity' was sometimes seen as part of their illness, especially for women. But in theory they gave up their sexuality – along with many other aspects of their humanity – when they entered the institution. In part this was to stop them breeding.

The desexualizing of the psychiatric 'inpatient' has left a legacy of neglect of people's sexual lives.

Some service users report that they do not get support with some of the dilemmas they may experience in relation to sexuality and relationships; or the treatment may get in the way.

'They prescribed me an antipsychotic drug, which caused me to be impotent. All of a sudden you can no longer perform. It's like a lightning bolt. And they don't warn you in advance.'   ('Jack', consumer, Washington DC, 1996)

Some psychiatric medication may also lead to less sexual pleasure for women (Mowbray and Benedek, 1990). Mowbray and Benedek comment that 'inpatients rarely discuss the effects of medication on their sexual functioning and more frequently therapists do not ask'. Prescribers need to start these conversations by informing people of the possible effects on sex, rather than expecting people to introduce what they may find a very difficult topic – and in any case they may have no idea that their sexual problem has anything to do with their medication.

Most service users – like most other people – have sex. One study found 73 per cent of women users interviewed had had sex in the last year (Mowbray *et al.*, 1995). Some may want to talk to mental health workers about relationships or sex. Others may not. Mental health workers need to provide opportunities without being intrusive. They need to be positive towards different types of relationship – lesbian or gay as well as heterosexual; unmarried as well as married; one-night stands as well as commitments – whilst recognizing that some people may need help to stop or change relationships that are damaging. It is clear that these standards are not always met:

'When I came out of the hospital I started to have therapy with a man at the day centre. When I talked to him about my (lesbian) sexuality he said "careful Stella, not so loud". I think that's bad – that's telling me to be frightened, and I am not going to be frightened any more.'   (Phillips, 1994)

'The new mental health commissioner was previously a Christian marriage counsellor. He told me he wanted to prevent schizophrenia by introducing more Christian counselling in the State mental health services'   (Consumer, US).

Whilst staff are entitled to their own religious beliefs they are not entitled to try to impose them on service users. The time of treating people with mental health problems as though they did not have a sexuality, or as though they should, childlike, take on the values of staff in developing their sexual choices, should by now be over. It is not entirely over, but it is time that it was.

Rape and assault

It is ironic that people for whom sex has historically been 'forbidden', have not been protected from rape and assault. A study in Ohio found that 60 per cent of women in a state hospital had been raped and 46 per cent otherwise sexually assaulted prior to their hospitalization; during their time as inpatients 47 per cent had been raped in the hospital by staff or other inpatients (Crossmaker, quoted in Mowbray and Benedek, 1990). Work in the UK – including media work by Esther Rantzen – has exposed the lack of safety from assault in many British psychiatric facilities and care homes.

The supposed invisibility of sex may help conceal assault: if sex 'doesn't happen', it may be easier to make out that sexual assault, including assault by members of staff, does not either. But assault is invisible mainly because people diagnosed mentally ill are powerless to make it known and stopped – as some abusers know all too well when they select someone to rape or abuse. There are almost insuperable barriers for anyone diagnosed mentally ill to being believed if they report such a crime (Blom Cooper, 1992; MIND, 1992).

It is imperative that mental health and criminal justice agencies take steps to prevent assault and to deal with it effectively if it happens. In Britain this means revising the Crown Prosecution Service's priorities on pursuing 'winnable' cases (i.e. those where witnesses are 'credible') (Women Against Rape and Legal Action for Women, 1995); offering women the choice of women-only space in mental health services; and introducing policies, training and user information on sexual harassment and abuse in mental health agencies (MIND, 1992).

Whether or not to have a child?

Women with serious mental health problems sometimes know little about contraception and, if they do become pregnant, they appear more likely than other women to do so in an unplanned way (Oyersman *et al.*, 1992). They might welcome above-average support with contraception, given Cook's finding that many find typical methods of birth control difficult. Some do not know their own bodies well and therefore may not feel comfortable with inserting a cap or IUD. Having the confidence to ask a man to wear a condom – a problem for many non-mentally ill women – may be harder for someone who is feeling anxious or depressed. And taking the pill regularly may be difficult for someone who has difficulty with planning and organizing her life.

The answer to this is not for mental health staff to start adding the contraceptive pill to the tablets given each night in the hospital ward without even discussing it, as happened to Ms Cox (Leighton Cox, 1988). Nor is it to encourage or persuade people to take an injected, long-lasting contraception without explaining the risks and alternatives. But mental health staff can offer to provide information and link people into the support they may want in order to make choices. The possible choices are numerous and highly individualized: a woman might decide to think through how she could realize an ambition to get pregnant. She might choose to have sex without penetration, or to take her partner to a family planning clinic to discuss condom use.

Cogan found that 65 per cent of the women she interviewed wanted to talk about contraception along with other issues of sexuality – for instance, 33 per cent wanted to talk about lesbian or bisexual feelings. Once a woman is pregnant she may be pressurized into having an abortion, on the now-familiar grounds that as someone with a mental health problem she should not have a child (Stefan, 1989). Conversely she may be pressurized into **not** having an abortion, because of the beliefs of those running the mental health service she is using. For example, some American psychiatric hospitals have policies against aiding and abetting abortions – a policy that lost one social worker her job simply because she called a cab for a service user who had herself arranged to go for a termination. In a case in Illinois, a woman who was an inpatient decided she wanted a termination and was deemed legally competent to make this decision. The hospital refused to give her a pass. Although she was a voluntary inpatient she could have been involuntarily committed if she had decided to leave against medical advice. She did not get her termination.

'One woman inpatient who was pregnant told me how the staff had reacted. In the same day one nurse had told her that it was wrong to even consider having an abortion; and another had said it would be totally irresponsible to go ahead with the pregnancy.'   (Consultant Psychiatrist, Chicago, Illinois)

Whether a person gets an abortion they want – or whether they are pressurized into having one that they do not want – may depend on the accident of the beliefs of members of staff. It also depends on the policies of individual institutions, where these exist. Stefan (1989) found only two States with policies on abortions for women in institutions. The New York policy sensibly stated that each inpatient has the same right to carry a pregnancy to term as any other citizen and the same right to abortion as any other citizen. This commitment to non-discrimination appears rare.

Whether or not women get contraception or abortion often depends not on their informed choice, but on other people's prejudices about whether they should have children and on other people's moral values about abortion.

Deciding whether to become and whether to stay pregnant is not just a matter of knowing the facts about contraception, or abortion, and saying yes or no. It is a choice made in a context. For women generally, that context might include the strength of her wishes to parent, other life options available – such as work, the views of her partner if any, availability of finances to care for the child, and the availability of help and support from other family members and friends. Many women with or without mental health problems get pregnant accidentally, or do not work out all these issues ahead of time, but once pregnant the context usually becomes highly significant. For women with mental health problems the context often has additional complexities.

Women may be concerned – or may be encouraged to be concerned – about genetic risk. In the UK genetic information appears sometimes to be used to discourage people from having children. In the US genetic counselling appears rare – as it is a health service that is not reimbursable under insurance programmes such as Medicaid – but this does not stop people picking up the idea that their children may be disabled. Often they pick up this idea in a highly exaggerated form. For instance:

'I've decided not to have children because my husband's illness (schizophrenia) is genetic. It would get passed on.'   (Jane, New Jersey)

'Sarah' was advised by her GP in Britain that she should not have children as she had manic depression and her children would be likely to have it too. Being scientifically trained she went and read the research for herself and found out that the risk was much smaller than the GP had implied. She now has two children.

Overstating genetics can also impact on family and spousal relationships. Oyersman et al. (1992) note that husbands sometimes give up on women who have a mental health problem, assuming that if they have children they also will be 'tainted'. One man in Washington DC left his wife when their son was diagnosed schizophrenic, on the grounds that he decided it was her genes, not his, that caused the problem. A DC woman diagnosed manic depressive told me of her family's resistance to her boyfriend because, as he was also manic-depressive, he was a risky genetic match. His parents felt the same way about her. These examples are the result, not of genetic counselling, but of bits of knowledge gained through the media. They are part of what is likely to be a growing pattern of genetic stigma and discrimination (Gostin, 1993).

Another part of the context concerns support. Some women may not have strong social networks, or partners (Mowbray et al., 1995). They may have had difficult childhoods themselves and not learnt much about parenting. Will there be anyone from mental health or other services to help prepare and teach them? Will there be anyone to look after the child if they have to go into hospital, or if they are not coping well at home?

A further context is legal. If the woman is not able to meet the high cultural expectation of looking after her child totally independently, what will happen? The answer of course is that she will probably be separated from the child, permanently or temporarily. A 'choice' between having an abortion and having a child whom you are likely to lose could accurately be described as Hobson's choice.

Then there is the question of what else a woman will do if she does not have a child. Some women may crave the valued role of mother partly because of an absence of other roles, like worker. Unemployment of people with serious mental health problems is variously estimated at between 70 per cent and 85 per cent in the US (Mancuso, 1993). Rehabilitation programmes have traditionally focused on finding work for men and often finding nothing for women (Williams et al., 1993; Nicholson and Blanch, 1994). Women need to be supported to take on a choice of roles, including both work and parenting. As Stefan puts it, 'these women are fighting to be seen as mothers in a society that still finds them unfit for any role at all except those arising from their labels' (Stefan, 1989). Sands (1995) found that low income women who had serious mental health problems and were caring for children saw parenting as making their life fuller – and may have found it one way to affirm their 'normalcy'.

Finally, pregnant women with mental health problems are often poor. They often have no antenatal care and do not eat nutritious food. They are prone to miscarriages (Mowbray et al., 1995). They may be worried that the drugs they are taking will harm the foetus – or conversely they may be encouraged to come off all medication for the sake of the foetus, which may cause havoc with how they themselves feel. They may live in housing that does not accept children and may as a result need to seek new accommodation. They have an awful lot to deal with.

After the birth

Some women lose their child in a legal sense before it is even born (Stefan, 1989). For some the child is taken as soon as medically possible (Perkins, 1992). Some women respond to this trauma by having more and more children: 'Mary has had eight so far – each time her latest baby is taken into care, she has another one' (Perkins, 1992).

After losing a child the parent often gets no support in dealing with the grief (Sayce, 1996). They may not want support from the services which they hold responsible for removing the child (Perkins, 1992).

Other parents keep custody and care for their child or children, often despite rather than with the help of the mental health services. For example:

'I was in the hospital on and off for over 15 years. I wasn't well and it was because of my political beliefs too. In the end I drove my car into the White House gates, I was so frustrated. I was put in the White House ward (the psychiatric ward for people who have committed crimes linked to the White House). The staff advised my wife to divorce me because of my illness. But we've stayed together, thanks to her and thanks to our faith in God. It was no thanks to the mental health services. They didn't give any help for my family. I'm back at home now, with my wife and my children.'   (Robert, Washington DC, 1996)

'My husband looked after my son when I was in the hospital. He was a very good father. I don't know what I would have done otherwise. No one ever offered any support.'   (Judy, Austin, Texas, 1996)

Many parents feel that their right to parent is tenuous. They are afraid that if they do the wrong thing, or become ill again, they will lose their children. For example:

'I only married so that there would be this image of normalcy . . . the issue was not just my mental illness . . . what bothered them was pointedly my promiscuity as they saw it, my relationships.'   (Cogan, 1993)

Whilst some therefore do not seek help at all, others underplay any problems they may be having.

Mental health professionals in the US have informed me of cases where women have nonetheless called services for help – only to have their children immediately removed and fostered, sometimes for months or years. In many cases an offer of help with the child at the point of crisis could avoid this eventuality. Resources have, however, increasingly been directed into the 'policing' aspects of risk assessment rather than into the supports that might obviate the need to police.

The lack of support is often debilitating. In both the UK and the US childcare is very hard to obtain without private funds. Even with money, in the UK in the early 1990s there were about nine day places for children under 5 years for every 100 born (Sayce, 1996). Most mental health services are not child-friendly. In the UK, in the absence of facilities where mothers can be admitted with their children, they may be admitted to general psychiatric wards, where staff may know nothing about childcare and other inpatients may object to the presence of a child (Sayce, 1996). These wards are also often not safe. The Mental Health Act Commission reported on one woman who stood like a sentry at her door to ensure the protection of her child (Mental Health Act Commission, 1993).

A cautionary tale

The only way to change this situation is to bring about systemic change. It is not enough just to give service users better information and 'choice' about contraception – although this is needed. They must have decent options to choose between. This means systemic change based on principles of non-discrimination and access.

Some cities and states have tried to create such changes. In 1992 New York State set up a special task force on the subject. They found that 16 per cent of children in foster care – some 10 000 children – had at least one parent with a mental health problem. The task force held public hearings, identifying problems ranging from fragmented services to lack of attention to children in mental health assessments (Blanch *et al.*, 1994). Then they started a process of change, based on clear recommendations including incorporating family concerns into all policies and procedures; developing self help and support groups; increasing supported housing for families; providing training for the family courts; and improving information for service users. Projects have been set up: for instance, a Resource Centre in the Bronx where hospitalized parents and grandparents can visit with their children, and an Orange County 'Invisible Children' project, offering supported housing, advocacy and crisis services. Parents with psychiatric disabilities have access to information: for instance, the leaflet *Helping Yourself Through the Family Court Proceedings, a Guide for Parents with Psychiatric Disabilities*, which gives suggestions on how to prepare for the court case; how to find peer support; how to plan care for the child in ways that are helpful and convincing to a judge; and how to explore different alternative outcomes, like open adoptions.

However, they sound a cautionary note:

'Administrators and service providers need to be prepared to encounter discriminatory attitudes, particularly from the press, but also from some providers. At times during the task force process it was implied or even stated that people diagnosed with severe mental illness should not marry or have children because they are too fragile psychologically, carry a genetic predisposition, or are incapable of providing a stable family environment.'

Systems change has to include influencing the media and tackling prejudices held by the public and by service providers. This was confirmed by events in Chicago.

Chicago is one of a small number of cities that has made serious efforts to address systemically the needs of parents with mental health problems and their children. Until the 1980s Illinois State law allowed termination of parental rights purely on the grounds of parental mental illness. The law was changed, thanks to an effective local advocacy campaign. As a result some parents with serious mental health problems were enabled to care for their children, sometimes with considerable support from the Mothers' Project. This project provides intensive support to parents and children in the form of a therapeutic day programme, outreach to parents and children in their homes, and help with loaning toys, securing benefits, work, housing, health care, contraception and more (Zeitz, 1995). Specialist hospital and outpatient services are also available. The components of a comprehensive service began to be articulated and developed (Miller, 1992).

Until the early 1990s, progress was gradually made in Chicago. Then, in 1992, a woman in a middle-class suburb, whose child had been fostered because of her mental health problems, had the child returned to her. She killed him, in a crime that became front-page local and national news. Editorials churned out the view that decision-makers were stupid to have allowed a woman with schizophrenia to have custody of a child. Following objections from local psychiatrists and others, the press did subsequently examine the social circumstances of the case in more detail. They did not, however, make any mention of the fact that other Chicago women with schizophrenia were successfully taking care of children.

Journalists often claim to achieve objectivity in their writing by 'balancing' two opposing viewpoints, thus supposedly pulling the piece to a neutral middle ground. On this topic, the view that a woman with schizophrenia might in some cases be able to look after a child – perhaps with support – does not feature at either end of the pole. It is not even on the extreme edge. It did not appear in the news coverage (although one letter from the American Psychiatric Association's Committee on Women's Issues was published).

Not surprisingly the case provoked huge concern, which led to some positive policy moves. Following recommendations from a specially formed task force, an interdisciplinary assessment team was set up to make recommendations to the court on the potential risks to the children of people with mental health problems. This team, which combines experts in psychiatry, psychology, child development and social work, makes assessments based on observation of parenting both at home and in the hospital – where previously assessment often meant prospective 'inkblot' type tests by psychologists who never even observed parent and child together. Child development, psychiatric and other assessments are also made. The team has trained judges in how to evaluate the evidence that might be put before them, including the inadequacy of prospective methodologies. The result, after a year of the team's operation, appeared to be improved quality of court decision-making (Dr Laura Miller, personal communication).

However, the team covers only a part of the city, deals with five or six cases at any time, and had a waiting list in 1996 of 60. Families normally only reach the team after children have been fostered – by which time their experience of the childcare services, where staff generally lack training in mental health, is likely to be investigation rather than support. Following assessment, the parent and child may be linked into some support, like the Mothers' Project – or there may be no support available, in which case lack of support may be seen as a risk factor. The team may have no option but to recommend continued separation between parent and child.

These difficulties could be solved by re-directing resources into support and childcare help, rather than spending most money on investigations and court cases. Once a child with special needs is fostered, the cost is approximately $900 per month. A court case might cost an additional $10 000. $900 per month could fund some intensive support, plus childcare, which in many cases would enable the parent to keep the child at home. Instead, if the parent seeks help when she is at the end of her tether, the greatest likelihood is that the child will be removed and fostered. By the time she is referred for help to the assessment team or the Mothers' Project, she may have gone through years of trying to get her children back from foster care. Mary Ann Zeitz, Director of the Mothers' Project, cites one case where by the time the woman was referred to the Project, the eldest child, aged 7 years, had already been in 37 foster placements and had been abused in foster care. In many cases such histories are avoidable.

Part of the reason they are not avoided lies with the media coverage of Ms Wallace, the woman who killed her child. Since this tragic case a backlog of cases concerning custody by parents with mental health problems has built up in the courts. For every one case resolved, a further six are going to court. Resolution has slowed down. Professionals interpret this as a response to fear of trial by media. In this climate of opinion every judge knows that if they err on the side of caution, by stalling or terminating parental rights, they are highly unlikely to face lawsuits or trial by media; whereas if they make one decision in a lifetime that means a child is hurt by someone with a mental health problem, their reputation will be on trial. There is little incentive to take even the most carefully planned risk. Many of the women who are awaiting an outcome in their case say that they feel they are being judged for the crime of Ms Wallace. Mental health funders continue not to fund services for these parents, perhaps partly because they shy away from a responsibility that could put their name, rather than that of childcare agencies, into the media spotlight if another story hits the press.

Since this case, the Mothers' Project has done some work with journalists to try to alter the climate of opinion in the media, with some limited success. Editorials on another case of death – probably a cot death – stated that there would always be an element of risk in child welfare and that a death did not necessarily imply wrongdoing (*Chicago Tribune*, 22 November 1995). Nonetheless, reports quoted experts questioning the wisdom of granting custody to someone who appeared inadequate, and gave little voice to anyone with a mental health problem.

It is not possible to create change for individuals without engaging in systemic change; and systemic change depends upon a climate of public opinion that allows decision-makers to do the unpopular – to allow people diagnosed mentally ill to care for children with support. The Mothers' Project has gradually moved into areas such as law and media relations, as well as therapy, in response to this need.

Even in Chicago, where such major efforts have been made to improve the service systems, equally major obstacles remain.

In the UK we are all too familiar with policy trends that derive from a single, atypical case. As Ms Wallace's case has slowed progress in Chicago, so the killing of Jonathan Zito in the UK prompted policy changes in adult mental health which were opposed by nearly every professional, legal, charitable and user organization in the country as unworkable and unethical (Sayce, 1995). Such cases become prominent because they resonate with strongly held stereotypes and fears: in the case of Jonathan Zito, his killer was a stranger, black and 'mad'. In communications terms, they fit with the dominant narrative, which is that people with psychiatric disorders are dangerous and need to be controlled. There is a sub-strand in this narrative which says that there is a particular risk to children – witness all the NIMBY (not in my back yard) campaigns against proposed mental health facilities based on the headline 'our children will not be safe' (Sayce, 1995).

Repper and Brooker suggests that these campaigns are becoming increasingly successful in stopping mental health developments in the UK (Repper and Brooker, 1996). It is highly likely that occasional cases involving harm to a child will become prominent again, including in the UK. They can make debate unbalanced and strangle the progression of policy and practice. They suggest forcibly that part of the work of improving opportunities for people with psychiatric disabilities to parent has to be a pro-active attempt to change the 'narrative' as well as to respond rapidly to inaccurate journalism. The new narrative needs to say that people with mental health problems can make good parents, or adequate parents, or bad parents – they are not uniform. It needs to portray their view of their experience and the view of their children. It needs to include comments like the one from David Leiker which opened this chapter.

In 1997 MIND held a conference in the UK at which a mother diagnosed with schizophrenia spoke about how she was bringing up her 9-year-old son. She had learnt to manage her voices, and her son understood this as 'you sometimes daydream, Mum'. An adult daughter talked of her pain at being permanently separated from her mother. She was told only that her mother was 'busy': in fact she was in a psychiatric ward, trying to make contact through letters and cards with her daughter – but the letters were never forwarded. These women talked on a number of radio shows and to the press: the taboo was beginning to be broken.

Conclusion

When the 'insane' and 'feeble-minded' were forcibly sterilized, the idea driving the programmes was that letting them breed might be expensive; might lead to crime and other social ills; and might taint the gene pool. All these ideas are alive and well and still influencing our policy and practice – although there are also other forces at play, like the pioneering work described here in Chicago and New York State (and in many parts of the UK; see Chapters 11 and 12). The risk to the next generation has been re-framed to include the risk of bad nurture as well as bad nature, and the methods used to control childrearing have changed from sterilization to discouraging pregnancy and terminating parental rights. Some of the new methods are less drastic than the old – but arguably terminating parental rights can be at least as traumatic as sterilization.

Part of the reason we have progressed so little is that the debate has been wrongly located. Most discussion of these issues focuses on the conflict between the child and the parent – or the conflict between the foetus and the parent – rather than on the broad social question of what value we place on disabled people and whether as a society we are prepared to pay for the support services they may need. Without debating social value, we leave in place the philosophical underpinnings of the sterilization programmes. These said that it was a social service to reduce the number of disabled people and the social burden they created. As a society we have not developed an alternative social vision. Still less have we created a 'narrative' in the public debate that conveys this vision to the public.

There are other reasons for lack of progress – for instance, the particular stereotype that people with psychiatric problems will harm children, the fact that rehabilitation and other mental health services have largely neglected women's needs, and with them parenting needs. But resolving these parts of the problem will not open up opportunities for service users to parent unless we promote a new social vision.

The bases for such a vision are principles of anti-discrimination and access. This approach makes a statement, that disabled people are valued by society equally with other people. Disabled children are valued – their birth is not discouraged. Disabled adults are recognized as potential parents, who may need support – perhaps intensive support – in order to give them access to the opportunity to be parents.

This change will take time. The fruits it could bring are a break from the tradition that brought us forced sterilization and so-called 'euthanasia'; and the beginning of a system that accords value to disabled people.

Acknowledgements

I would like to thank all the service users and mental health professionals in the US and the UK who shared their views and experiences with me. I am also indebted to the many writers referenced here who have pioneered work on these issues, especially Susan Stefan who, to my knowledge, was the first to look comprehensively at rape, reproductive rights and parenting rights for women diagnosed mentally ill.

Risk assessments of infants born to parents with a mental health problem or a learning disability

Lucy A. Henry and R. Channi Kumar

Mother and Baby Units are hospital-based services for mentally ill mothers and their young infants. They generally serve three, somewhat overlapping, functions (Kumar *et al.*, 1995): (1) the treatment and rehabilitation of mothers who develop acute post-partum illness; (2) the treatment and rehabilitation of women who have a history of pre-existing mental illness and who have recently had a child; and (3) the assessment of actual or potential risk to infants within the context of maternal mental illness and associated problems. As Kumar *et al.* (1995) point out, these clinical facilities are very rare outside the UK, Canada, Australia and New Zealand, yet there are no clear theoretical opinions either for or against them which explain their widely differing approaches. There is a lack of research on the effectiveness of Mother and Baby Units in terms of maternal recovery and also little direct experimental evidence on how maternal mental illness may affect child outcome (Kumar and Hipwell, 1994).

The purpose of this chapter is to discuss some of the ethical issues which arise when specialist Mother and Baby Units are asked to carry out parenting assessments. These involve a judgement as to whether the mother is able to care for herself and her child both physically and psychologically, now and in the future. The Children Act (1989) (Williams, 1992) dictates that the welfare of the child must be paramount, and whether the child's welfare is best served by keeping him or her with the natural mother, given the mother has a mental impairment or a mental illness, is sometimes a very difficult decision.

At the Bethlem Royal Hospital Mother and Baby Unit, a parenting assessment usually necessitates a 6-week inpatient stay by the mother and her baby, during which time her parenting skills are assessed by a multidisciplinary team. Many difficult issues and judgements come up in the area of parenting assessments, and the following sections outline some of these difficulties. First, the complexities of assessing parenting skills are discussed in the context of some of the ethical issues. Next, we discuss the assessment of infant development and the bearing this may have on maternal behaviour. Finally, we consider parenting in two particular areas, mothers with learning disabilities and mothers with schizophrenia, briefly reviewing the research evidence on parenting in these groups of mothers and illustrating the general ethical points that can arise with case histories.

These two areas are chosen because they present particularly difficult dilemmas in many cases. However, we acknowledge that many of the same points apply to other disorders and depression is one of the most researched areas in the field (e.g. Murray, 1992; Murray *et al.*, 1996; see also Kumar and Hipwell (1994) for a general review of the effects of maternal puerperal psychiatric disorder on infant development).

Assessing parenting

Assessing what constitutes 'good enough' parenting is very difficult, and many authors have commented on the fact that parenting remains a very difficult construct to measure because of its complex multidimensional quality (e.g. Mrazek *et al.*, 1995). Different cultures have different childrearing practices, as do different subcultures and social classes. However, most of the research into parenting and developmental psychology is Western and middle-class in orientation. This means that assessing parenting in families who are not Western or middle-class is open to many biases which even enlightened professionals may find difficult to identify. It is also possible that higher standards are applied when assessing parenting in the context of parental mental illness because professionals know that their recommendations must be able to withstand legal scrutiny if there is a conflict of interest (Ramsay and Kumar, 1996).

These broad issues form the backdrop for the assessment of parenting. Added to them are the particular orientations of the professionals involved, the strategies they use to carry out the assessments, the interpretation of the information and their willingness to draw firm conclusions about the adequacy of parenting (Budd and Holdsworth, 1996). Given the high stakes – possible separation of parent and child – it is imperative that professionals are aware of the potential biases that may emerge and work to avoid them.

In a recent review article, Budd and Holdsworth (1996) outlined a general framework for assessing what they refer to as 'minimal parenting competence'. They point out that although general descriptions of good parenting are available, including constructs such as warmth, nurturance, acceptance and responsivity, on the whole we lack ways of measuring them. Even where measures are available, many are not well validated and most are not developed to assess the lower limits of parenting competence. This leads to problems because there are no behavioural indicators of minimal standards in parenting, let alone norms for the relevant range of parenting skills. In addition, research-based assessment of parenting looks at parenting on a continuum, whereas in the clinical setting an all-or-nothing decision must be made at one particular point in time using the information available. Budd and Holdsworth (1996) argue that professionals assessing parenting are left to rely on personal experience, on subjective clinical impressions and on instruments designed for assessing optimal parenting. It is at this point that the dangers of middle-class bias and other forms of bias emerge. A further problem is that by looking in detail at parenting in a particular case without reference to appropriate norms in a reference population, higher standards than are reasonable may be expected. The effects of examining parenting in detail are also likely to affect behaviour. Some parents may be impaired by constant evaluation, others may present themselves in an overly favourable light. Either way, the problem remains of generalizing to the home situation (Ramsay and Kumar, 1996). The supportive yet judging relationships between professionals and families may also prevent parents from making the best independent use of their own resources. The mere fact that a professional has come in alters the family situation and could lead to the development of dependent relationships and affect the parents' perception of their parenting role.

In order to provide the most comprehensive and fair assessments of minimal parenting competency, Budd and Holdsworth (1996) suggest that assessments should cover eight dimensions: historical information about previous behaviour; intellectual functioning; adaptive and social functioning (e.g. social risk factors such as unemployment and social isolation); personality and emotional functioning (including any psychiatric diagnoses); parenting knowledge, attitudes and perceptions (using well-researched and validated instruments); parent–child interactions (using direct observations); child functioning (cognitive, behavioural, health, emotional adjustment); and parental responsiveness to previous interventions (whether positive or not). They also suggest that assessments should explicitly focus on parenting strengths and weaknesses, and point out that given the lack of consensus about minimal parenting standards, professionals should adopt a conservative stance when interpreting the information.

A similarly comprehensive approach is advocated by Gopfert et al. (1996) in relation to parents with mental illness. They suggest that the following broad headings should form the basis of any assessment: (1) parenting, including capacity to provide a stable and nurturing environment for the child's physical, emotional, social and intellectual needs, and including checks for evidence of abuse; (2) the mentally ill parent, including level of disturbance, sense of responsibility, use of help and symptoms which impact on parenting directly; (3) the other parent (where relevant), including commitment to maintaining the family, attitude to the illness of the partner and health/emotional resources; (4) the marriage (if relevant), including the ability to communicate and work together plus any history of conflict or violence; (5) the child, including developmental progress, attachment status, unusual characteristics and available outside relationships; and (6) the context and extended family, including support from others, financial and housing status and environmental stress/life events. This approach stresses the importance of seeing the family in its wider context before judgements of effectiveness of parenting are made, acknowledging the complexity of the task whilst pointing out that the final judgement is necessarily a subjective one.

Herbert (1996) has also produced a guide for assessing children in need and their parents. He notes several key factors in the assessment of parenting including having clear objectives; using methods which are comprehensive, fair, practical, ethical, accurate and relevant; and keeping the child's wishes in mind if he or she is able to express them. Herbert (1996) outlines a list of six areas which should be evaluated: parental knowledge and attitudes to parenting; parental perceptions of the child's behaviour; the quality of parenting; observations of parent–child interaction; the quality of the attachment of child to parent; and parental emotions and responses to stress. Many of these areas are similar to those reviewed earlier, but the guide is not specifically tailored for assessments of parents with a mental illness.

In the context of Mother and Baby Units specifically, a promising measure of parenting sensitivity has been described by Hipwell and Kumar (1996). The Bethlem Mother–Infant Interaction Scale (BMIS) is based on nurses' ratings of the quality of mother–infant interaction and has been used clinically to examine whether nurses' ratings are predictive of the eventual outcome of a parenting assessment. Initial findings were that BMIS ratings differed across different diagnostic groups and that ratings made in the second week of admission were strongly related to whether eventual separation was recommended. This suggests that the BMIS may represent one method of detecting difficulties in the mother–infant relationship early on and could eventually lead to possible interventions to prevent separations. However, the BMIS was designed for use with mentally ill mothers and scores were highly skewed when measures were taken of the interaction of dyads where the mother was not ill.

Black (1990) points out that parents may differ with different children such that parenting is effective with one but not another. This underlines the need to consider parenting in the context of particular children in the family, because child factors such as disability or difficult temperament may affect the conclusions. In addition, parents may be effective with children of one age and less effective with children of another age. Realistically, parenting assessments are unlikely to reveal direct evidence on how a parent may cope in the future with a toddler when the assessment examines parenting of a young infant. However, these issues are extremely important for the welfare of the child. A further problem is that decisions made at the point of discharge from a Mother and Baby Unit will in many cases remain unaltered, even if the mother's functioning improves or declines later on (Ramsay and Kumar, 1996).

In the UK, the Children Act (1989) requires that the welfare of the child must be paramount when courts are making decisions, and that delay should be avoided as it is likely to prejudice the child's welfare. However, decisions made at one point may not reflect the developing picture, and it is, practically, very difficult to incorporate potential for the improvement in parenting over time. The converse, the potential for 'significant harm', referring to ill-treatment or the impairment of health or development, is also hard to assess. Black (1990) points out that predicting future behaviour is notoriously difficult, and that demonstrating that any harm suffered is related to the standard of care is also difficult. This perspective, taking the welfare of the child as most important, raises ethical issues with regard to the mother as well. Removing a child from his or her mother may produce significant distress for the mother. Evidence suggests that mothers who have given up their children for adoption continue to think about them for the rest of their lives (Rynearson, 1982). Whether this could affect the course of an illness is open to debate, as is any position which suggests that a child or infant who cannot give consent could help to provide a 'normal' experience for a mother (Ramsay and Kumar, 1996).

The general effects of parental psychiatric disorder on children have been reviewed by Hall (1996). They include increased risks of psychiatric disorder (the contribution of both genetic and environmental factors is acknowledged) and direct risks including infanticide, child maltreatment and insecure attachment status. There are also a multitude of factors which contribute to the child's resilience or vulnerability including constitutional factors (e.g. intelligence, gender, prenatal adversity), perpetuating factors (e.g. separations from the mother, sociocultural factors and family functioning) and precipitating factors (e.g. life events and current family psychopathology). Hall (1996) makes the point that, given the risks to children of parental psychiatric illness, it is vital for professionals to assess and treat families as skilfully as possible.

Many of the issues raised in relation to parenting assessments become even more difficult when the child in question is an infant. The next section considers some of these difficulties.

Looking at child outcome – the special case of infants

Most parenting assessments will consider whether appropriate developmental stages are being reached. Cognitive development has typically been seen as particularly important amongst child development theorists, but emotional health and development, social development, mental health and physical health are equally important. In most parenting assessments, a very brief cross-sectional glimpse of the child is obtained, so it is difficult to look at developmental progressions. However, current functioning can be compared to population norms and predicted achievement to obtain some idea of progress (e.g. motor milestones, cognitive development).

There are, nevertheless, special difficulties in assessing developmental progress when the child is still an infant. This is, by definition, what is required in Mother and Baby Units, and the assessments must take place within a relatively short time-period. Monitoring of health, feeding, weight gain and physical development can take place relatively easily and can be checked against developmental norms. Assessments of cognitive and motor development can be carried out using standardized instruments such as the Bayley Scales of Infant Development (Bayley, 1969), but their reliability, particularly for very young infants, is very variable (McCall, 1983). Therefore, there is a question as to whether a meaningful developmental quotient can be obtained in infancy.

However, assessments become even more difficult with respect to the mental health and emotional development of the infant. Zeanah et al. (1997) point out a number of problems in this area. Firstly, there are very few measures of psychopathology in infancy, and even fewer recognized disorders, although research is increasing rapidly in this area. As our knowledge stands to date, any number of factors may increase risks for a variety of later conditions, and any particular deficit in the first 3 years may relate to a number of different possible outcomes in terms of later psychopathology. This means that we can rarely predict likely outcomes with any specificity, and it is particularly difficult to disentangle a large number of risk factors which may include mental illness or mental impairment in the mother. The best current thinking is that the greater the number of risk factors, the greater the concern. When a Mother and Baby Unit is asked to recommend whether separation of mother and baby is in the best interests of the child, it is necessary to assess how far the mental illness or mental impairment may contribute to or exacerbate a constellation of other related factors. It is also important to check the child's health to exclude congenital disease, brain damage etc., which may affect its contribution to mother–infant interaction and, thus, bear indirectly on perceptions of the mother's responsiveness and sensitivity.

A second major problem with identifying signs of psychopathology in infants is that, even if we could delineate reliable indicators, they are very likely to change during the first 3 years, a period of rapid and far-reaching change and development in the child (Zeanah *et al.*, 1997). This means that in a typical parenting assessment which lasts a few weeks, we have the problem of a very limited time-frame as well as a lack of understanding of what exactly to look for.

A final issue with respect to child outcome is the attachment relationship he or she has formed with the mother. Since Bowlby's work on attachment (Bowlby, 1969) the importance of a secure attachment relationship during the first 3 years for later development has rarely been questioned. Black (1990) emphasizes the need to take a developmental perspective when considering separations. Young infants and older children are less at risk from separation because they have either not yet formed attachments or have learned to maintain relationships in the absence of the attachment figure.

An explicit aim of parenting assessments where mothers and babies are admitted together is to try to maintain the continuity of this relationship and avoid attachment disruption. This is particularly important once the infant reaches 7–9 months, when consistent preferences for certain caregivers are expressed and distress occurs upon separation from caregivers (Schaffer and Emerson, 1964). When an assessment spans this age range, the ethical issues become very difficult. To keep the infant and mother together for another several weeks when eventual separation is likely could be harmful to the infant – it may affect his or her ability to form a new attachment to another caregiver and the separation may cause undue distress. However, to separate infant from mother during this period may be equally harmful if the final decision is to keep the two together. Even where one places the welfare of the child foremost, the dilemmas remain.

With very young infants where attachment relationships are in the process of being established, research is less clear about the effects of separation. Certainly, infants of this age show little overt distress and stranger wariness, but we cannot rule out adverse effects of changes in caregivers before 7–8 months. Infants of only 2 months respond negatively to the 'blank face' of their mother or asynchronous interactions with their mothers (Murray and Trevarthen, 1985). It is a general observation that infants reared by multiple caregivers may be 'overly' sociable, but the long-term effects of this are not clear. In cases of institutional rearing up to the age of 4 years, behavioural and emotional difficulties are more common (Tizard and Rees, 1974; Hodges and Tizard, 1989).

To date, there is little research linking the clinical disorders of attachment (e.g. ICD-10, DSM-IV) to research classifications of attachment (e.g. secure, insecure, disorganized) developed using the Strange Situation Procedure (Ainsworth *et al.*, 1978). These classifications have been used extensively in developmental research over the past two decades. However, although they are not clinical divisions, there is evidence of better outcomes for securely attached infants in terms of cognitive and social development (e.g. Londerville and Main, 1981; Sroufe *et al.*, 1983; Slade, 1987). Higher proportions of insecure and disorganized attachment relationships are found in infants of mothers with psychiatric disorder (e.g. Hall, 1996). This implies that poorer outcomes may be associated with maternal mental illness. Insecure and disorganized attachments are unlikely to indicate clinical levels of symptomatology in most cases, but further research on clinical disorders of attachment in infants of mothers with others forms of mental illness or mental impairment is needed given that the risks of insecure attachments are likely to be elevated.

Recently, Hill (1996) has raised the issue of the parent's attachment to the child, something much neglected in attachment research. He argues that a secure attachment relationship is most likely to develop when the parent shows 'commitment' to the child. This is defined as 'the way in which parents give priority to, and refuse to give up on, their children' (Hill, 1996, p.8). The parent's contribution to the attachment relationship is characterized by varying levels of commitment as well as other features including preoccupation with the child's well-being, continuity in parental behaviour towards the child, provision of a caring and secure base for the child and awareness of the child's needs. Hill (1996) discusses how these factors may be threatened by the same processes which make the adult susceptible to psychiatric disorder in the first place, such as social disadvantage and poor experiences of their own parenting. He also suggests that they may be affected by the illness directly. For example, preoccupation and sensitivity to a child may be reduced if the parent's mind is filled with delusions and abnormal beliefs. This approach offers a promising insight into how the attachment of the parent to the child may be assessed to give a complementary picture of reciprocal attachments between parents and children.

Ethical issues in practice

Next, we will discuss some of these methodological and ethical issues in relation to two particular types of maternal disorder: first, in mothers with a learning disability; and secondly, in mothers with severe mental illness, taking schizophrenia as the example. These two areas are chosen because they illustrate the tension between the rights and welfare of the child and the rights and well-being of the mother in cases where the decisions are particularly difficult. They illustrate the point that in many cases 'there is an inherent conflict of interests between the mother's wishes and the child's needs' (Kumar and Hipwell, 1994).

Parenting and learning disability

In the first part of this century, questions arose as to whether those with a learning disability should be allowed to bear children at all. In general, the response was 'no', given fears that excessive fertility in the mentally retarded would lead to ever larger numbers of children similarly affected (see Chapter 5).

More recently, it has been acknowledged that those with learning disabilities have as much right to bear and raise children as anyone without a learning disability. Certainly, more and more people with learning disabilities are having children.

However, concerns over the adequacy of parenting have now become the focus of attention. In accepting the parent's right to have children, consideration needs to be given to the position of the child and whether that child receives 'good enough' parenting. In the UK, social services departments often refer mothers with learning disabilities for an assessment of their ability to parent their babies. We have already discussed many of the difficulties inherent in providing such an assessment. How is this manifested if the mother has a learning disability?

Research on parenting by those with learning disabilities is conflicting, marked by both optimistic and pessimistic evaluations. Dowdney and Skuse (1993) reviewed the available evidence and concluded that part of the conflict may be explained by varying definitions of parenting competency and differences in the samples (e.g. some studies include women with IQs over 70; some consider only those referred already because of concern over the child's development). Further problems with the research comparing samples of parents with and without learning disabilities include failing to match for social class, very small sample sizes and brief observation periods. Tymchuk (1992) adds that much of the information we currently have is based on research carried out during a more restrictive time where bias against those with learning disabilities was common. In addition, the focus of the questions asked was more on parental 'inadequacy' than adequacy. Finally, given the complexities of parenting, it is not surprising that there is a lack of empirically established methodologies for assessing its adequacy in parents without learning disabilities, never mind amongst those with them.

Dowdney and Skuse (1993) argue that there is general agreement that IQ does not relate systematically to parenting ability unless it falls below the level of around 55–60. Thus, in many cases, IQ alone cannot be considered a bar to effective parenting. However, it has been found that the proportions of children with learning disabilities are higher amongst parents with lower IQs. In a comprehensive epidemiological study, Reed and Reed (1965) found that in the general population of parents with normal intelligence, 1 per cent of children had moderate to severe learning disabilities. This rose to 15 per cent where one parent had a learning disability and 40 per cent where both parents had a learning disability. Given that raising a delayed child is more stressful, often requiring higher standards of care and attention, many learning disabled parents may have a more difficult job in the first place. There is certainly more work required in tracing the genetic transmission of specific disorders or syndromes from parents to children (e.g. Laxova et al., 1973). However, this is not applicable to every parent with a learning disability. What emerges from the research is that regression to the mean occurs with the majority of children of those with learning disabilities falling within the range of mild learning disability to normal intelligence (see reviews by Tymchuk, 1992; Dowdney and Skuse, 1993). Therefore, it is at least as important to look at various characteristics of the child, including what types of special or additional care the child may need, as to look at the capabilities of the parent. IQ level alone is never sufficient. This is only one of many complex factors. One of the key difficulties is that, amongst parents with learning disabilities, low IQ is often only one of a number of psychosocial disadvantages they suffer. For example, significant proportions of a sample of mothers with learning disabilities in Sweden (Gillberg and Giejer-Karlsson, 1983) were from the lowest social class (13/13); were unmarried (12/13); were living in a socially underprivileged area (11/13); received social security help (8/13) and had deprived childhoods (8/13). Therefore, it is very difficult to separate whether a learning disability on its own makes parenting difficult, or whether, as seems more likely, a learning disability together with a number of other risk factors reduces the scope for effective parenting. It is well established that the risk of abuse is heightened in the general population with respect to a number of factors including parental history (e.g. abuse), family make-up (large numbers of children, single parenthood), social context (deprivation, low socioeconomic status) and characteristics of the child (temperament, learning disability, psychiatric disorder).

In fact, there is very little research comparing parents with learning disabilities with parents matched for background, living circumstances and socioe-conomic status, let alone more sophisticated research which also attempts to take into consideration the characteristics of the children as well and look at directions of causality. It is also necessary to look at parenting of children of different ages to assess whether parenting can be more or less effective at different stages of development. As demands grow on the parent, this may increase the risks of a breakdown in parenting. Most assessments are cross-sectional and give us little information about developmental changes.

Application of middle-class standards or standards which would not generally be applied to those without learning disabilities is also common and has been commented on by several authors (e.g. Gath, 1988; Tymchuk, 1992). Tymchuk (1992) points out that although there is evidence that mothers with learning disabilities show differences in their interaction with children as compared to middle-class mothers (less varied, less supportive, less reinforcing, more punitive and directive), it is not clear whether this applies only to mothers with low IQs living in poverty. In addition, there is no necessary single standard of parenting in Western cultures which dictates that one style must be regarded as inherently more valuable than another. Parents with learning difficulties are also more likely to come to the attention of services in the first place, and we have little by way of appropriate norms with which to compare them. Therefore, further research is needed which compares mothers from similar backgrounds, in similar circumstances, with similar children but who vary in intellectual ability, in order to tease out the risks of intellectual and other forms of disadvantage. Interestingly, in one study of decision-making abilities of mothers with and without learning disabilities where social class and circumstances were matched, no differences were found (Tymchuk et al., 1990). More generally, Tymchuk (1992) summarizes the capacity of mothers with learning disabilities to learn, maintain and generalize parenting knowledge as similar to that of other parents living in poverty.

Therefore, in assessing the parenting of mothers with a learning disability, care must be taken to look at all of the relevant factors. Current research is limited, but does suggest that a learning disability need not be a bar to effective parenting.

Case example

Ms B was a 19-year-old single woman referred for a parenting assessment with her 3-month-old baby. She had a borderline learning disability (IQ 70), limited literacy skills and had not, apparently, lived independently successfully since leaving home at the age of 16 years. Her family were not supportive and records showed a history of social services involvement throughout Ms B's childhood. Ms B had had a short relationship with the father of the baby, but he was not involved with the baby in any way and little was known of him other than that he was in his 50s, married and may have lived near Ms B's parents.

Ms B appeared to be very attached to her baby and viewed him as the most important thing in her life. She was able to learn the practical aspects of caring for her baby with guidance from staff. However, observations of her parenting revealed that she was not able to offer consistent care, emotional contact and stimulation. Even though it was felt that she had the skills, her organization was poor, and whilst no physical harm had come to the baby while in her care, staff on the Unit felt that this was a risk when Ms B was unsupervised.

The child's welfare was paramount and it was felt that Ms B had significant unmet emotional needs of her own which interfered with her care for her baby. She often placed her own needs above those of the baby. However, the learning disability was not a major issue. Ms B was able to learn how to care for her baby and to learn about safety issues. She also had sufficient knowledge and understanding to be an effective parent. It was her social circumstances (lack of support) and her emotional needs which were seen as the root of the problem. In this case, the decision was to recommend foster care for the baby.

This decision took away the 'right' of the mother to care for her child because it was felt that the welfare of the baby would not be catered for adequately by his natural mother. Given the range of risk factors involved, including lack of a supportive partner, it was felt that Ms B did not have enough resources to overcome them. Questions can be raised as to whether the standards applied were too strict and whether the needs of the mother were ignored. Ms B disclosed to one member of staff that she might take her own life if she lost her baby, but the seriousness of this threat was unclear. However, even when such threats are serious, they cannot affect the decision, only the way the mother is supported afterwards. If the decision to separate mother and baby had been made earlier (the baby was over 4 months when the separation took place), this could have been better for the baby and fairer to the mother, but, equally, it may have been hasty to recommend separation before Ms B had been given a reasonable chance to learn parenting skills. It was felt by the team that the learning disability was not relevant, but it is impossible to say whether there was some underlying bias against Ms B because that label had been attached to her. These issues are, ethically and morally, very complex. They also involve predicting future behaviour and assuming that Ms B would not, in the near future, acquire effective enough parenting skills to care for her child. No actual failure of parenting had occurred (e.g. abuse or neglect), but it is very questionable as to whether one should wait to see if this happens and put the child at risk, although it is likely that past behaviour is the best predictor of future child abuse (Tymchuk, 1992). The final decision had to assert the child's interests over the mother's. Unfortunately, this meant that despite the fact that it was clear that Ms B had significant emotional needs, yet another blow was dealt to her by separating her from her baby.

Parenting and schizophrenia

There are several ways in which having a schizophrenic illness may affect parenting. Goodman and Brumley (1990) suggest three possible routes: (1) passivity and social withdrawal on the part of the parent; (2) delusions which may involve the child; and (3) exposure of the child to the incongruent affect often associated with schizophrenia. Seeman (1996) describes several other common features of mothers with schizophrenia. She argues that many mothers avail themselves of less adequate prenatal care. They may also have difficulties with intimacy and negative symptoms (e.g. apathy, lethargy) which can be exacerbated by neuroleptic medication. Socialization may be limited in the home and thus hinder the child's interaction with other children, and perceived fears may result in rituals or eccentric protective measures. Communication between the parent and the child may also be affected by the disorder, as schizophrenia often causes disturbance in communication.

Kumar and Hipwell (1994) point out that there may well be differences between the negative and positive symptoms of schizophrenia in relation to child outcome, and that research generally does not reflect this heterogeneity. In their review of the literature on the effects of schizophrenia on parenting, they noted findings of less sensitivity in mothers with schizophrenia, less social contact, poorer performance by infants on tests of object constancy at age 1 year, as well as conflicting findings concerning whether there were raised levels of insecure attachment when the mother had a diagnosis of schizophrenia.

In reviewing the evidence concerning the effects of parental psychopathology on parenting, Goodman and Brumley (1990) came to similar conclusions: parenting was less reciprocal, little responsive and less involved in general. However, they pointed out that there was little research looking specifically at mothers with different diagnoses than mothers with psychopathology in general. In their own study, Goodman and Brumley (1990) compared parenting in mothers with schizophrenia, mothers with depression and well mothers all matched for demographic characteristics (predominantly black, low income and lone parents). In general, schizophrenic mothers showed the lowest scores on the measures of quality of parenting. For example, they demonstrated the least affectional involvement and responsiveness to their children; the childrearing environment provided by schizophrenic mothers was significantly poorer than that provided by well mothers; and the mother's diagnosis accounted for significant portions of the variance in some measures of child outcome (the children were aged 3 months to 5 years and significant effects were found for IQ and expression of appropriate affection and annoyance). However, Goodman and Brumley (1990) point out that it is the quality of parenting which is the key factor, not diagnosis as such. While a diagnosis of schizophrenia does not necessarily mean that parenting is ineffective, it appears to have more of an impact on parenting quality than a diagnosis of depression.

This finding was backed up in a recent survey of 100 admissions to the Bethlem Royal Hospital Mother and Baby Unit. Kumar et al. (1995) looked at the proportion of cases in which the team recommended that the mother be separated from her baby at discharge. Comparing mothers with diagnoses of schizophrenia ($n = 20$), affective psychosis ($n = 56$) and non-psychotic disorders ($n = 24$), separation was recommended far more often in cases where the diagnosis was schizophrenia (50 per cent as opposed to 8 per cent in affective psychosis and 4 per cent in non-psychotic disorders). Kumar *et al.* (1995) noted that the primary source of risk in mothers with schizophrenia was neglect 'because the mothers were unaware, lacking insight or unable to concentrate and sustain consistently safe behaviour' (Kumar *et al.*, 1995, p.19). Therefore, in clinical practice, it does appear that the lower quality of parenting is being reflected in more decisions to separate mothers from their infants.

Rogosh *et al.* (1992) attempted to integrate the multitude of factors which affect parenting, including the supportiveness of the social network, the physical living environment and the temperament of the child, with parental diagnosis, self-esteem and perceptions of one's own parenting experience. Mothers with schizophrenic disorders, schizoaffective disorders and affective disorders were studied and path analysis was used to try to examine the links between these factors and parenting attitudes. Frequent relapse (an index of severity) related to parenting attitudes relatively independently. Other current factors showing direct and indirect links to parenting attitudes included emotional support and self-esteem. The historical factors concerning the mother's own parenting were also linked to parenting attitudes and these included close relationships in childhood, a history of childhood separation and loss, and maternal laxness/uninvolvement. This study underlines the fact that parenting attitudes are multiply determined and suggests that severity of illness may be relatively separate from the other factors involved. Nevertheless, the total sample was relatively small ($n = 48$) and further research is required before firm conclusions can be drawn. An additional problem with these studies is that most use very different measures of parenting quality and the reliability and validity of many parenting measures can be severely questioned (Budd and Holdsworth, 1996).

In summary, most of the research evidence does suggest that parenting quality may be impaired in groups of schizophrenic mothers. However, more research teasing out the effects of illness from other adverse circumstances is required. Each case must be assessed on its merits as the following case example illustrates.

Case example

This case was also discussed by Ramsay and Kumar (1996).

Ms A was a 41-year-old woman with a 4-month-old baby. A parenting assessment was requested by social services. Ms A had a 16-year history of paranoid schizophrenia and cooperated intermittently with antipsychotic medication. When well, she showed no behavioural abnormalities, but during relapses she became hostile, deluded, paranoid and unpredictable. Ms A had one other child aged 7 years with whom she had no contact. Ms A had known the baby's father for under a year and he was dependent on alcohol when they met. They sometimes fought violently and Ms A had taken out an injunction against him. However, since that time, the baby's father had undergone detoxification, his relationship with Ms A had improved, and the injunction was being revoked.

Early in the pregnancy, Ms A had stopped taking her medication and as a result her mental state began to deteriorate. Staff were very concerned about her by the time of the birth. She was aggressive and hostile, and rough with the baby. Therefore, the baby was removed into foster care pending a parenting assessment. However, on admission to the Mother and Baby Unit, Ms A's mental state was normal and she was insightful into the fact that she had a chronic mental illness requiring medication. Over the 8-week assessment, Ms A gradually became more relaxed with her baby, made good eye and vocal contact and was comforting and affectionate.

Because no perceived risk to the baby was observed, the team decided to recommend that Ms A return home with her baby at the end of the assessment. However, several caveats were included. It was felt essential that monitoring and support of Ms A and her partner in the community by mental health, primary care and social services was provided. The baby was also placed on the local child protection register. Finally, any resumption in drinking on the part of the baby's father or a decline in Ms A's compliance with medication were both regarded as likely to affect parenting adversely. As with the earlier case, a consideration of the resources available to help Ms A cope, given the risk factors, formed the basis of the decision.

This case illustrates that decisions which at one point favour separation can alter at a later point in time if circumstances change. The main factor operating in Ms A's favour may have been her compliance with medication and the opportunity to learn parenting skills in the supportive atmosphere of the Mother and Baby Unit. However, one weakness of the assessments discussed in an earlier section is that they do not see parenting in the 'real life' situation where support and advice is not available 24 hours a day.

There is also the difficulty of defining 'significant harm' within the scope of the Children Act (1989). Literally, it is meant to be taken as ill-treatment or the impairment of health and development (Adcock, 1996). The literature suggests that there are effects of having a parent with a mental illness, and more severe illnesses appear to lead to more marked effects (e.g. Hall, 1996). However, this is not necessarily the case for every parent with a mental illness, and the effects may not constitute 'significant harm'. Increasing the likelihood of insecure attachment is one possible effect of a parent with a mental illness, and can be included as constituting grounds for 'significant harm' (Adcock, 1996). But, increased risk of insecure attachment may also stem from the mother working full-time outside the home in the infant's first year (Belsky and Rovine, 1988) and this is rarely regarded as grounds for doubting parenting ability. Therefore, although the literature on parenting by mothers with severe mental illness gives some markers for possible long-term effects, the clinical team is still left with a decision about an individual case for which group findings may not be particularly relevant.

The outcome in this particular case was to keep mother and baby together, but with careful monitoring and compliance with medication. Whether the impetus to carry on taking medication on the part of Ms A and to cease drinking on the part of the baby's father for the good of the baby would continue can only be guesswork and in the absence of clear evidence to the contrary, a team decision is likely to favour the optimistic viewpoint. This may be in the interests of both mother and child, but one argument might be that the position of the baby is somewhat precarious. A question remains as to whether the baby is in any worse position than a similar baby from a similar social group in similar circumstances. We are rarely able to answer this type of question clearly. Whether the mere fact of a diagnosis of schizophrenia biases professionals against keeping mother and baby together is also an open question.

Conclusions

There are many difficulties with parenting assessments which range from the methodological to the ethical. This chapter has discussed some of the issues which arise in the context of parenting assessments on a Mother and Baby Unit. Several key points have emerged. First, there are no clear standards for 'good enough' parenting, or reliable methods of measuring parenting, although some researchers are beginning to work on comprehensive assessment packages. Second, there are particular difficulties in assessing infants' development in the context of adequate parenting. For example, assessing psychopathology in infancy is particularly problematic. Third, we are making decisions about possible separation of mothers and babies during the critical first year during which attachment bonds are forming – mistakes may be very far-reaching for the infant. Fourth, a learning disability on the part of the mother is no bar to effective enough parenting and all factors must be taken into account. Despite this, having a learning disability is often associated with other social disadvantages which impact adversely on effective parenting. Finally, in the presence of severe mental illness such as schizophrenia does often mean that clinical teams opt for separation. However, individual cases vary considerably and every case must be looked at carefully on its merits. Overall, the assessment of parenting is a complex and multifaceted endeavour which must be recognized fully by those with clinical responsibilities for making recommendations about the separation of mothers and babies. Many of the ethical issues which arise centre around placing the welfare of the child first and overriding the mother's wishes.

Postnatal depression in the context of changing patterns of childcare: the implications for primary prevention

John L. Cox

Introduction

The subject of this chapter was chosen because of my greater awareness that parental perinatal mental disorder may have serious consequences for young children and that parenting in a 'post-modern' society is particularly difficult and at times very stressful. I also wished to encourage debate about the benefits and disadvantages of the changes in family life over the last 40 years, and the impact of these changes on the prevention of postnatal mental disorder.

The children of the 60s, whose parents were studied by Pitt (1968), brought up their children in a different family context from their own parents, and with less available family support. The nuclear family according to many commentators (see Neuberger, 1994) has been reshaped by changing attitudes to sexual intimacy and contraception, as well as by uncertain durability of longer term relationships, including marriage. This cultural shift is reflected, and reinforced, by the media and in particular by television (Starkey, 1996). The nuclear family has indeed been radically changed by sharp increases in the divorce rate (one in four in the UK), postponed marriages and childbearing, as well as by cohabitation, smaller families, step families and dual-earner marriages. These trends are similar to those occurring in the US where Acock and Demo (1994) report that only 71 per cent of children lived with two parents compared with 88 per cent in 1960, and that at least a quarter of children lived with a single parent compared with only 9 per cent 30 years ago. As conception is intimately linked to the nature of the relationship between the parents, and the mother is regarded as the primary caregiver in most societies, understanding the effect of changing family structure on perinatal mental disorder, and of changing attitudes towards childbearing, is essential.

This chapter has been revised from a Plenary Lecture delivered at the Biennial Meeting of the Marce Society, London 1996. It was also published in full in *Archives of Women's Mental Health* **1**(2), 1998.

It is of interest that the family is described by international writers (United Nations, 1994) as a 'pivotal institution' from which societies continue to derive strength, and forge their future. Many such families are also faced with additional crises such as famine, poverty, unemployment, drugs and AIDS, as well as the impact of new 'wage earning life-styles'. Desjarlais *et al.* (1995) have discussed evidence for the adverse effect of these misfortunes on family life and particularly on economically marginalized children. Rosenfield (1989) argued that role overload and subsequent low power for women may explain their greater frequency of anxiety and depressive symptoms when compared with men.

In many Western countries however these changes are occurring alongside another social revolution with wide implications for the family; mental health services are provided 'in the community' with the closure of mental hospitals and an expectation that the mentally ill are cared for by their family. Thus the family, now under siege, is expected to assume more, rather than less, responsibility for the health of its members, and especially for those who suffer from mental disorders.

In a national survey of 100 child death reviews carried out by Falkov (1996), there was evidence of psychiatric morbidity in the family in 32 cases and evidence that the perpetrators were mentally ill in 25 cases. Marks and Kumar (1995) found that the greatest risk to the life of an infant was in the first year. An infant is four times more at risk in the first year than in other years of life from being killed by its parents. Furthermore the Confidential Inquiry Report into homicides and suicides by mentally ill people (Royal College of Psychiatrists, 1996) found that over 20 per cent of mentally ill perpetrators were mothers with a depressive disorder. These findings demonstrate the need for a fully resourced perinatal psychiatry service including a mother and baby unit. Prettyman and Friedman (1991) found that only 20 per cent of Health Districts had a designated Mother and Baby Unit and although specialist perinatal day hospitals, such as the Charles Street Unit in Stoke on Trent (Cox *et al.*, 1993; Boath *et al.*, 1995), reduce the need for admission and have considerable advantage compared with primary care (Boath *et al.*, 1999), these day hospitals do not always prevent admission, especially when there is risk of harm or when a 24-hour community service is not in place.

There is however at the present time greater recognition of the need for clinicians and researchers to make public the policy implications of their research with regard to perinatal services and the effect of perinatal mental disorder on children. It is also appropriate to increase awareness of the evidence for adverse effects of separation and divorce on the mental health of children (Ayalon and Flasher, 1993). Murray and Stein (1989), used data from their studies which found adverse effects of postnatal depression on infant development. Others have drawn specific attention to the public policy implications of such knowledge, and of the need to be more firm advocates for improved resources.

Similarly the advocacy of the Marcé Society is beginning to influence government policy, through its members in the UK and with particular effect in Australia, with regard to improved primary care screening for PND. Several Australian states, for example New South Wales (Commonwealth Department Human Services and Health, 1994), have produced proposals for a community perinatal psychiatry service using the Edinburgh Postnatal Depression Scale (Cox *et al.*, 1987), and made cogent recommendations about appropriate treatment strategies in primary care. A needs-led perinatal mental health service is now more likely to be acknowledged as a priority by health authorities in the UK; the recommendations for commissioning such services by the Royal College of Psychiatrists (1992) were most timely.

Sociocultural perspectives

The perspective of social anthropology for an understanding of the causes and consequences of childbearing mental disorders is particularly apposite and relevant when considering the requirements of a needs-led service. Thus, childbirth **is** a 'Rite of Passage' which cannot be restricted to a discrete localized life event like a burglary or the death of a pet, or even to an unwanted house-move. It is a staged social transition which includes separation, liminal and reincorporation phases, and establishes a different valency of relationships between parents and a secure environment for infant learning and development. Price (1995) has speculated that parenting behaviour has been facilitated in evolutionary terms by neuro-hormonal mechanisms, including the effect of oxytocin and prolactin which maintains mothering behaviour such as maternal/infant proximity. Is it possible that new parenting behaviours now being selected by an evolutionary process will ultimately modify further these neuro-hormonal mechanisms?

Fitzgerald (1995) has argued that the transmission of parenting skills is impeded by 'breaks' in knowledge transfer between generations. Her paper 'Cultural breaks in women's knowledge' presented at the Marce Meeting in Sydney in 1995 was most relevant to these considerations. Fitzgerald argued that such 'breaks in knowledge' are caused by the migration of a daughter from her family and in particular her mother (as experienced by Cambodian refugees), as well as by delayed childbearing and by smaller families, and that it is the lack of this knowledge transfer from parents which leads to lowered self-esteem and clinical depression.

Cultural competence is indeed of particular importance when training health professionals in the perinatal field and facilitates sensitivity to the way in which cultural values and attitudes are transferred between mother and infant. Such competence is necessary for an understanding of the presentation of postnatal depression especially in ethnic minority communities such as the Punjabi-speaking Sikh community in Wolverhampton (Clifford *et al.*, 1997), as well as for women from a majority subculture such as the Potteries in Staffordshire. For example, Murray *et al.* (1995) found that these women were more likely to be depressed if they gave up work 'reluctantly' or had a poor relationship with their mother.

Clinical and research priorities

What is the relevance of these contemporary changes in family structure, and in particular the increased rates of divorce and separation, for the recognition and management of postnatal depression?

It is already established, though not often emphasized, that women with young children are more likely to become depressed if they do not have a confidante, intimate partner or husband. This early finding of Brown and Harris (1978) has since been replicated in the USA (Weissman *et al.*, 1988), and more recently in the UK (OPCS, 1995). This latter study found that lone parents, and those living alone or without close relatives, were more likely to experience neurotic symptoms than other women, and that people living in couples with no children were the least likely to have mental health problems. Having children increased the prevalence of psychiatric symptoms and especially irritability. Living in a one-person family was particularly associated with increased alcohol and drug dependence (OPCS, 1995). It is known that a single first-time mother is at increased risk of being admitted with a puerperal mental illness within 30 days of delivery (Kendell *et al.*, 1987).

In comprehensive reviews by O'Hara and Zekoski (1988) and Boyce (1994) dysfunctional marriages (marital problems, partner hassles) were causes of PND, as well as secondary consequences. In only one study reviewed by O'Hara and Zekoski was no such association found. However, there are no studies as yet to determine whether these marital problems lead on to separation or divorce. RELATE counsellors, however, are aware that these events do occur in the immediate postpartum period; Dominian (1968) referred to this special possibility in his influential book on marriage breakdown. It is likely that research in this field will be particularly important. A hypothesis of an increased frequency of separation and divorce in the peripartum period could readily be tested.

It is of considerable interest that in most of these studies the marital difficulties had occurred in the setting of untreated postnatal depression. It is not known the extent to which these marital problems would have been ameliorated or not occurred at all if the depression had been identified and fully treated. Clinical experience suggests that this latter strategy would prevent family break-up.

Prevention

Bearing in mind the above considerations, what are the implications for the prevention (primary, secondary and tertiary) of perinatal mental disorder – and of postnatal depression in particular? Although there is evidence for increased rates of depression over recent decades in Sweden (Hagnell *et al.*, 1982) and in cross-national comparisons (Cross-national Collaborative Group, 1992), there are no studies to establish whether or not the rates of *postnatal* depression have increased. A replication of Brice Pitt's study of postnatal depression would therefore be extremely pertinent at the present time. It is a most plausible hypothesis that the frequency of PND – incidence and prevalence – is increased because of the changes in social support and in particular by the present lack of continuity of family relationships. It is also possible that changes in the nature and duration of marital relationships would partially explain the greater interest in, and concern about, postnatal depression compared with 30 years ago – at least as determined by the present levels of media interest and by the increasing number of research reports and popular books.

It is probable therefore that useful generalizations can be made about the prevention of perinatal mental disorder, and several possibilities come to mind, e.g. ensuring that education about parenting responsibilities and the stages of child development are more widely available, or revising the curricula of parent-craft classes to take into account the impact of reduced family support and increased vulnerability to depression and the anxiety of women who are single because of separation or divorce.

There is a need for greater availability of premarital counselling, and for health education in schools with an emphasis on the culturally appropriate core family values relevant for a multi-faith society. The benefits of encouraging greater expectation of enduring marital relationships, and ongoing responsibility for the care of children could be more emphasized in primary prevention programmes, as well as making family planning clinics and sex education programmes more available. More provision of nursery facilities at the workplace, and adequate welfare supports would help also to reduce the prevalence and personal impact of postnatal depression.

Secondary prevention of PND by early screening and making available advice to parents who experience relationship strain secondary to depression will assist to break the 'vicious circles' which maintain such depression (Figure 7.1).

Early intervention using treatments of PND known to be effective (e.g. counselling and antidepressants) is more likely if education packages designed by general practitioners for general practitioners are developed and if specific training for primary care-based community psychiatric nurses and health visitors continues to be provided.

Attempts to recreate more culturally appropriate postnatal 'routines' to enhance parental self-esteem and to affirm core tasks of parenthood could also be considered. For example a review of the nature and content of the postnatal 'visit' and deliberately enhancing professional and lay support, would increase the value of such routines and provide 'structure' to the postpartum period which Western society has largely lost. Churches might also consider a more popular, yet secular, Naming Ceremony to emphasize for parents the importance of their infant and of their family responsibility even when they are in a reconstituted family. Such a ritual might facilitate the provision of more informal social support from neighbours and friends.

Figure 7.1 'Vicious circles' in the origins of postnatal depression

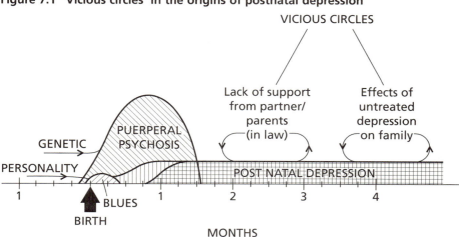

In this way the advantages of new family structures, and of more diverse parental responsibilities, could become apparent and the disadvantage of post-modern families diminished. The Marcé Society, which provides persistent peer review and encourages academic and clinical endeavour, may have to consider further these wider public health responsibilities.

There **is** a need to respond to an earlier challenge of Aubrey Lewis and to determine more precisely the effect of parental mental disorder on family structure and understand more fully how adverse effects are ameliorated.

'For the Sociologist the family is a nuclear unit; for the anthropologist, bonds of kinship are of the first importance; and for the psychiatrist the family is the matrix within which the individual is moulded and developed, the area where his strongest emotional ties are formed, the background against which much of his most intense personal life is enacted. There is, therefore, a need to study the family, not only from the psychoanalytical and psychological standpoint, but also to discover how mental illness impinges upon it, and what effects this sort of incapacity has on the family structure.'   (Lewis, 1956)

Postnatal depression adversely effects family structure and function and may lead to unwanted divorce or separation. One of our tasks I believe is to prevent as far as possible these and other adverse consequences of perinatal mental disorder, which readily impair parenting ability and lead to a transmission of disadvantage to the next generation.

Working with parents with mental health problems: management of the many risks

Alison Beck-Sander

Under UK law, the Children Act 1989 (Department of Health, 1989) leaves us in no doubt that the needs of the child are paramount in all Children Act court proceedings where a conflict of interest arises between parent and child. Adult and child services must act in accordance with the child-centred philosophy behind this Act. Nevertheless services do sometimes come into conflict. It is the aim of the first part of this chapter to explore some of the factors which may give rise to these conflicts and to then consider some possible solutions. The second part of the chapter focuses on the particular risks associated with parents with mental illness, written from an adult forensic perspective.

Conflicting perspectives

The Children Act (1989) places the needs of the child in the foreground. Section 1(1) of the Act states that 'when a court determines any question with respect to the upbringing of a child . . . *the child's welfare shall be the court's paramount consideration'*. By contrast, the Mental Health Act (MHA) 1983 (Department of Health, 1983) considers both the mental health needs of the adult and matters of public safety. Therefore an admission for assessment, for example, under Section 2 of the MHA requires that the patient 'is suffering from a mental disorder of a nature or degree which warrants detention . . . and that he ought to be so detained *in the interests of his own health or safety or with a view to the protection of other persons'*. These statutes guide service provision and direct the thinking of service providers. Although the Acts are not incompatible with each other, the perspectives they engender in service providers may conflict with one another because one focuses attention on the needs of the child and the other on the adult, albeit in the context of the risk they pose to others.

The political climates in which services operate can vary enormously depending on government policy and media focus. Services also exist in different social and cultural climates which give rise to differing risk priorities. For example, in the context of a forensic service, where many inpatients have committed serious offences such as multiple rape or homicide, the risk posed by an individual who threatens to hit someone may be considered minimal. The risk may be taken far more seriously by a busy social services department if the individual who is doing the threatening is a parent, and the person who is being threatened is a social worker attempting to supervise contact with a vulnerable child.

Services also have different working practices and terms and conditions of employment. This variation can lead to vast discrepancies in outlook. For example the risks posed by an individual, Mr R, may be perceived very differently by workers in the following different settings:

Worker A is required to visit Mr R on his own at home. Mr R lives on a run-down housing estate on the edge of town. A has heard that Mr R hit a colleague and broke his nose. He does not know what will happen if Mr R attempts to hit him. He is concerned for his personal safety and for the fact that he cannot afford to take any time off work. A is also concerned that Mr R may pose an immediate risk to his own children. A is unclear about the implications for himself if he falsely decides that the children are not at risk and something later happens to them.

Worker B is required to interview Mr R in an alarmed interview room at her place of work. She has been able to inform her colleagues of the potential risk posed by Mr R and is assured that if needed they will come to her aid within minutes. B is clear about safety procedures at her place of work and she is aware that her employer will support her if Mr R attempts to assault her. Similarly, B feels comfortable that if she follows practice guidelines and properly documents her reasoning for believing Mr R's children not to be at risk, her employer will support her even if her decision turns out to be wrong.

On the basis of these two examples it is clear that worker A is more likely to perceive that Mr R poses a risk (both to his children and to A himself) than worker B even though the material facts of the case do not differ. Working practices can radically influence subjective decisions about risk because they affect how safe an individual feels in their job.

Conflicts arise in practice when services operate according to different working practices and service procedures, because the subjective element of the risk appraisal will be affected. These conflicts are further exacerbated by the differing focuses of child and adult services arising from their respective guiding statutes. In addition, the different social and political climates in which services operate may differentially influence their risk assessments and bring services into conflict with one another.

Overcoming conflict

Several approaches may help to reduce these conflicts between services. The need for improved multi-agency communication and transfer of skills and knowledge has become something of a platitude, albeit one which remains essential. One way of improving communication might be to agree upon realistic risk management goals.

First of all, a fundamental caveat of all risk management work is that all the risks posed by parents to their children cannot be prevented. At best risks can only be reduced. It is not even feasible to aim to *identify* all risks. Any service which adopted this aim would be doomed to failure. Furthermore its workers would be over-cautious in their risk assessments in a vain attempt to avoid any possible harm occurring. As risk is sometimes unpredictable, harm would eventually occur and in this event the workers would be vulnerable to scapegoating because the service would view the occurrence of harm *necessarily* as a service failure. Furthermore such a service would also be unable to work effectively with other services because of its unrealistic expectations.

Public education is a second factor which may be very important in overcoming conflict between services. Reducing risk cannot mean avoiding all possible risk. This brutal fact is difficult to swallow and should not encourage complacency when risks *are* predictable. Nevertheless the general public needs to be educated not to expect services to be able to avoid all harm. We cannot. If the public has unrealistic expectations about safety, then scapegoating is likely to occur when harm, inevitably, occurs. For example, when cruel child killers hit the headlines the public demands an explanation for their crimes. The media often attempts to pin the blame on social services, the police and other agencies for not having identified the killers sooner. This may give rise to conflicts both between and within services as attempts are made to allocate blame. Scapegoating can destroy staff morale and undermine good practice. These conflicts cannot be reduced until the public accepts that some risks are unavoidable and that sometimes no service or individual is blameworthy.

Is the goal therefore that services should attempt to avoid all *predictable* or knowable risk? Even this goal is highly questionable. A third factor in reducing conflict between services is recognition of the fact that there are often benefits associated with measured risk-taking. Many risks incur the potential for considerable benefits as well as the potential for harm. For example, allowing an incestuous child molester to return home to live with his family probably incurs risks associated with re-offending. Nevertheless after successful treatment and the development of a careful relapse prevention plan these risks may be considerably reduced. Furthermore there may be benefits for both the offender and his family from reunification. Some children blame themselves for the break-up of the family after abuse is disclosed. Many miss their abuser who may, in other respects, have much to offer the child. It may be important for the psychological development and welfare of the child to have a reformed parent return home, thus illustrating that it was in fact the parent, not the child, who was responsible for the abuse.

The task of risk management is therefore to carefully weigh up the harms and benefits in a risk calculation. Nevertheless this is another source of potential conflict between services. What may appear a 'reasonable risk' (i.e. benefits outweigh harms) to one service may appear unreasonable (i.e. harms outweigh benefits) to another.

Finally Carson (1994) draws attention to the importance of safe management structures to enable reasonable risk-taking. He describes three important components of safe management:

- Provision of a risk-taking policy to guide high quality risk decisions and to guarantee support if the terms and procedures of the policy are followed.
- Provision of a safety policy to minimize the likelihood of injury and information to employees about what to expect if injury does occur.
- Taking responsibility for staff training and for ongoing monitoring of service provision to ensure that standards of working practice are maintained.

Carson (1994) argues that service employees cannot be expected to make safe risk calculations if they are not safely managed. Furthermore, conflicts will arise, as argued above, between services operating with more or less safe management structures.

Mental illness and risk

The Mental Health Act (1983) defines mental disorder as 'mental illness, arrested or incomplete development of mind, psychopathic disorder and any other disorder or disability of mind'. It is worth noting that an individual will not be considered to be suffering from a mental disorder under the Act solely on grounds of 'promiscuity or other immoral conduct, sexual deviancy or dependence on alcohol or drugs'. The term 'mental disorder' is therefore a broad one. However, it does not necessarily encompass all behaviours which, if displayed by a parent, may lead them to pose a risk to their children. Furthermore for the purposes of the remainder of this chapter, I will focus on parents with *mental illness* as opposed to other types of mental disorder. Clearly many other mental disorders increase the risk posed by a parent to a child, e.g. substance abuse disorders, anxiety disorders, eating disorders, obsessive-compulsive disorders etc. These problems may coexist with a mental illness. However, co-morbidity aside, they are not explored further in this chapter.

What is mental illness?

Mental illness presents an enormous challenge to risk assessment because of its highly variable course. As a result the risk posed by parents to their children may vary considerably over time. It is therefore useful to distinguish acute and chronic mental illnesses. Acute illness is characterized by delusions, hallucinations and thought disorder. Whilst these may also be present to some degree in chronic illness the latter is more often characterized by a reduction of function: affective flattening, apathy and poverty of speech. After the first acute episode of mental illness, the course of the illness over the life-span tends to follow one of four general patterns.

First, the symptoms may resolve completely and never come back. Although free of mental illness these individuals may continue to be haunted by their experience of psychosis for some time. There is evidence to suggest that a variety of secondary problems may arise as a subjective reaction to the experience of psychotic decompensation and hospitalization, including secondary depression (e.g. Siris, 1991; Koreen *et al.*, 1993) and post-traumatic stress disorder (McGorry *et al.*, 1991). The risks posed by such individuals to their children are therefore complex.

The second mental illness profile involves repeated recurrence of psychotic symptoms with full recovery each time. Once again these individuals are at risk of developing secondary problems, however there is evidence to suggest that these problems are most apparent in earlier episodes of illness and at earlier age of onset (e.g. Mino and Ushijima, 1989). Overall people who experience psychotic illnesses have an increased risk of suicide which is around 10 per cent (Miles, 1977). This risk is generally held to be highest after a second episode.

The third pattern is a persistent defective state which becomes more pronounced after each successive period of acute illness. These individuals are, of course, not exempt from the aforementioned risks, namely depression, post-traumatic stress disorder and suicide. However, these secondary problems, if they develop, do so alongside a chronic mental illness profile.

The fourth and final pattern involves a progressive downhill course from the first psychotic experience. These individuals simply never recover from their first period of acute illness and their mental illness takes a chronic course. Nevertheless their symptoms may vary considerably in nature and severity over the course of their lives.

The proportions of individuals in each of these four loose categories depends on the definition of mental illness which is adopted. However, approximately 50 per cent of individuals who experience psychotic phenomena follow the first two patterns and 50 per cent the latter two (Ciompi, 1980).

People's experiences of mental illness are as different as the people themselves. No two individuals have the same experience of mental illness. There are many types of symptom, from delusions to hallucinations, from apathy to elation, from thought disorder to thought withdrawal. Each symptom may be interpreted in any number of ways depending on individual factors such as personality, intellectual ability, social and physical environment, concomitant difficulties, culture etc. It can therefore be very difficult to anticipate the risks posed by an individual with mental illness unless specific idiosyncratic details are known. Two cases illustrate the point.

Mr X has a long-standing mental illness which is prone to recur every 1–1.5 years. He is a deeply religious man from Jamaica. Even when he is not acutely ill he believes that he is a prophet who can communicate directly with God. This belief is to some extent supported by a local religious sect which he regularly attends. When he becomes acutely ill he hears the voices of angels and experiences tactile hallucinations which he describes as 'the spirit of the Lord' moving inside him. He also becomes elated in mood.

His psychiatrist is usually notified of his deterioration by either his wife or a work colleague. Mr X has worked as a night watchman with the same company for 17 years with only a few brief hospital admissions. He does not think that he has a mental illness but he is compliant with medication because he does not like going to hospital. Mr X has no convictions and the risk he is considered to pose to others is minimal.

Mr Y has a long-standing mental illness and is a polydrug abuser. In particular he says he uses alcohol, cannabis and cocaine on a regular basis 'with friends'.

However, Mr Y is becoming increasingly isolated. He has no regular contact with family and few consistent friends. He has not worked for over 10 years and has spent a considerable portion of the past decade in hospital. In the community Mr Y leads a chaotic lifestyle. He often fails to pay his rent and has ended up on the streets or in night-shelters on many occasions. When he becomes acutely ill Mr Y tends to feel 'full of energy' which he burns off by going for long walks and smoking cannabis. When he is walking he feels he is being followed. He also tends to believe that a government ethnic cleansing programme has sent individuals to seek out and eradicate 'undesirable' black men like himself. On several occasions he has been arrested by the police for offences ranging from being drunk and disorderly to causing grievous bodily harm and carrying an offensive weapon.

What risk of violence do people with mental illness pose?

Whilst high rates of mental illness have been found amongst fatal child abusers (Falkov, 1995), there are at least two points to bear in mind before jumping to premature conclusions on the basis of such data. First of all the absolute risk posed by people with mental illness is small (Mulvey, 1994). The statistics may therefore be distorted because a few individuals may pose a very serious risk to their children. It does not follow that all people with a mental illness pose a risk to their children.

Factors which place an individual who does not experience mental illness at risk of harming his or her children are equally relevant to individuals who do experience mental illness. Most importantly a history of abusing children in the past remains the gold standard amongst established predictors. However age, gender, poverty, criminality in the family, poor parenting, childhood experiences of abuse etc., are all predictors of risk which are as relevant in the mentally ill as in the non-mentally ill population. The relative risks associated with these various factors are largely unknown.

The most recent research shows that mental illness *is* a risk factor for violence in the community (Swanson *et al.*, 1994). Furthermore a combination of mental illness and substance abuse disorder significantly increases the risk of violence (Mulvey, 1994). Increased risk of violence is specifically associated with acute symptoms and when particularly active symptoms are controlled for, the association with mental illness in general dissolves. The particular symptoms which have been linked to violence are described as 'threat-control-override' (TCO) symptoms (Link and Stueve, 1994). TCO symptoms are said to have occurred when an individual has felt one of the following:

1. 'your mind was dominated by forces beyond your control';
2. 'thoughts were put into your head that were not your own';
3. 'there were people who wished to do you harm'.

When is this risk unacceptable?

The risk posed by a parent to a child may be difficult to quantify. The Children Act (1989) requires that a court be satisfied that certain 'threshold criteria' are met before making a care or supervision order in respect of a particular child as laid out in Section

31(2) of the Act: 'A court may only make a care or supervision order if it is satisfied (a) that the child concerned is suffering, or is likely to suffer, significant harm; and (b) that the harm . . . is attributable to (i) the care given to the child not being what it would be reasonable to expect a parent to give *him* (i.e. that particular child given his or her particular needs); or (ii) the child's being beyond parental control'.

According to Section 31(9) of the Children Act (1989) harm is defined as 'ill-treatment of the impairment of (physical or mental) health or development'. This harm must be attributed directly to parental care or to parental failure to prevent harm.

Having satisfied the threshold criteria, it remains within the power of the court *not* to make a care or supervision order. The court will consider the plans of the local authority and balance whether the parent can meet the child's needs against the likely outcome for the child of the planned local authority intervention (e.g. a foster care placement).

There are a number of ways in which a parent with a mental illness may pose a risk to their child, depending on their experience of their illness. Whether or not these risks meet threshold criteria must depend on assessment in individual cases. Some mentally ill parents may withdraw from social contact. In so doing they limit the opportunities available for their children to learn to socialize and to develop sources of support outside the family. The latter can become particularly important for the child if they remain with their parent when the parent's illness becomes active.

In situations where parent and child are socially isolated there is a danger that a highly dependent relationship may develop in which the parent places inappropriate demands and responsibilities upon the child. For example:

> Mrs D lives alone with her 12-year-old son. She has a relapsing paranoid psychosis and becomes extremely anxious when she is ill. At these times she often prevents her son from going to school or to visit his friends without her. When she accompanies him she has a tendency to express beliefs which embarrass him. Her son, therefore, prefers to try to look after his mother at home and to avoid contact with the outside world as much as possible.

Features of some mental illnesses, particularly chronic illnesses, are similar to those of depression, for example, apathy, passivity, disinterest and distractibility. Children may be at risk of parental detachment and neglect. Parental depression may be manifest as insensitivity and unavailability to the child which in turn may provoke anger and distress in the infant (Cummings and Davies, 1994). Research shows that depressed mothers have particular difficulties managing distressed infants (Cox, 1988). Furthermore insecure attachments may render a child more difficult to parent. The literature suggests that depressed mothers are more likely to resort to coercive and inconsistent parenting strategies. They are also more likely to avoid confrontations (Cummings and Davies, 1994). Children of depressed parents are at risk of a failure to thrive because of chaotic meal habits, parental irritability and difficulty controlling the children (Cox, 1988).

Greater risks to the child are associated with acute symptoms because of loss of contact with reality, as the following example illustrates.

Mrs S is a single parent caring for two young children with little social support. She has a relapsing schizophrenic illness. In the past she has had delusions that her children are angels who do not require earthly sustenance and must be protected from the evil world by being locked in a cupboard for several days (without food). She is normally compliant with her medication which eradicates her delusions. However she remains prone to periods of depression and poor self-image. In an effort to lose weight and improve her self-image she has recently been non-compliant with her medication resulting in a re-emergence of her belief that her children are possessed. Mental health professionals caring for Mrs S do not want to admit her to hospital because she is willing to accept medication as an outpatient. Concerns remain, however, about the risk she poses to her children.

The risks posed by a parent with a mental illness to their child are probably greater if acute symptoms of illness do not remit, as the parent may be unable to pay sufficient attention to the needs of the child. Particular concerns may arise if the child becomes incorporated into the content of a parent's delusional beliefs, as the previous example highlights. Over a prolonged period of illness delusional beliefs may become increasingly systematized and the meaning of the symptoms more coherent to the parent. The concept of 'rationality-within-irrationality' was coined by Link and Stueve (1994) and describes the notion that despite the irrational content of delusional beliefs, if it is accepted that they are experienced as real by the mentally ill individual, then it becomes possible to understand why that person should behave in a violent manner. In other words understanding the meaning an individual associates with their symptoms helps to explain why they behave as they do and how they are likely to behave in the future.

Junginger (1990) looked at the circumstances in which people act on commands from hallucinated voices. He found that individuals who experience 'hallucination – supportive delusions', in addition to their voices, and individuals who 'recognized the voice' were at greater risk of acting on their voices. It may therefore be important to ascertain the content of any hallucinated voices in case the individual is experiencing commands to commit dangerous acts. The research findings remain equivocal as to whether the dangerousness of the behaviour which is commanded is relevant in determining whether or not individuals will act on voices. Several studies suggest that individuals are more likely to act in cases where the commands are judged to be less dangerous (Chadwick and Birchwood, 1994; Junginger, 1995). However, other studies have found the dangerousness of the command to be irrelevant (Junginger, 1990; Rogers et al., 1990).

The association between the threat-control-override (TCO) symptoms, mentioned above, and violence, suggests that the child may be at particular risk of violence from the parent if the symptoms into which the child is incorporated are TCO symptoms. For example:

Mrs J believed that her eldest daughter, Sarah, was able to put evil thoughts into her mind. Sarah was the only child born to Mrs J from her violent first husband. Sarah was born with moderate learning difficulties and made many demands on Mrs J's time and patience. Mrs J believed that Sarah wanted to make her harm her other children. She attempted to strangle Sarah using a dog's lead. The child was placed in long-term care away from her mother. The other children remained with their mother who was not considered to pose a significant risk of harm to them.

To summarize therefore, when assessing the risks posed by a parent with mental health problems to their child, the following factors are worthy of consideration. First of all, the pattern of the illness. Do the symptoms remit? Second, the nature and meaning of the parent's symptoms. Are delusional beliefs symptomatic? Are there TCO symptoms? Is the child incorporated into these beliefs? Are there command hallucinations? Is the child implicated in the commands? Third, has the parent perpetrated dangerous behaviour in the past (particularly in response to acute symptoms and particularly to their child)? Fourth, can the parent monitor their illness and alert services if necessary? Fifth, is the parent compliant with treatment? Is treatment effective? Is hospitalization necessary? Six, is a support network available to the child, most importantly are other safe caregivers available? Can they monitor the situation? Finally, how responsive is the parent to the child's needs?

Conclusions

When assessing the risks posed by a parent with mental health problems to their children the perspective of the service provider can be crucially important in determining their conclusions. Legal statutes direct adult and child services to focus on the sometimes divergent needs of their different client groups. Furthermore, services develop different working practices, management structures and risk priorities which affect their risk assessments and may bring them into conflict with the assessment of providers of other services. Four strategies have been proposed in order to overcome these conflicts:

1. the setting of realistic risk management goals;
2. public education about the limits of risk assessment;
3. the importance of balancing harms and benefits when making risk calculations;
4. the need for safe management structures to facilitate safe risk-taking.

Assessing the risk posed by parents with mental health problems is a complex task which depends on an understanding of the nature and meaning of the symptoms for the individual, an estimation of the likely consequences for their behaviour and an assessment of the situational supports available to weather the storm. The perspectives of different service providers will all provide crucial contributions to the overall assessment and management of risk.

Understanding the needs of children and families from different cultures

Annie Yin-Har Lau

There are major associations between parental psychiatric illness and childhood disorder. The child is at risk of exposure to an accumulation of negative events, both acute and longstanding, which interact with the child's ongoing development and can lead to impairment of that child's physical and psychological growth. These children have a significantly increased risk of psychiatric disorder (Richman *et al.*, 1982; Rutter and Quinton, 1984). It is important in assessing the likely risks to the child that we undertake an integrated assessment of the mental health needs of the child, parents and family. This should address the strengths and vulnerabilities of the family, including the tensions in the interface with the professional system. This chapter also specifically considers how ethnocultural issues impinge on assessment and management.

Meeting with the relevant professional network

It is useful to start by meeting the key players in the professional system. The following questions need to be considered. Who is the assessment for, and to what purpose? What tensions already exist in the professional network? What is the view of the different agencies and institutions currently involved in the child's life – the school, health visitors, GP, Community Child Health, Local Authority, Guardian-*ad-litem*? Do they have different and conflicting experiences of the family? In the author's experience, professional tensions are commonly focused around the following areas

– issues of race and cultural relevance;
– professional judgements around the relative degree of risk to the child;
– what should constitute 'best practice', in order to safeguard the interests of the child and family.

These differences in the professional system may mirror or accentuate existing conflicts in the family system. It is well known that highly disturbed individuals and families have a tendency to involve a whole range of professionals, 'multi-agency families', who unwittingly maintain the abusive behaviours in the family (Dale *et al.*, 1986; Schuff and Asen, 1996). It is important for the child psychiatrist not to get drawn into a position where his or her assessment is likely to be disqualified at the outset. It is useful to be briefed if possible by all interested parties and to remain independent of partisan views, and to clarify what questions may help to resolve areas of professional disagreement, so that this can be covered in the assessment. This helps to maintain professional neutrality.

Family assessment

The most important question to look at here is the extent to which the parent's illness organizes and distorts adult and family functioning. It is known that the high rates of disturbance in these children are directly related to the associated psychosocial disturbance in the family, i.e. hostility and aggression, persistent marital discord and family disruption (Rutter, 1982). Direct risks to the children may include child abuse and neglect, and sometimes death, particularly for newborns of mothers with post-partum psychoses. It is a challenging task, however, for a mental health worker to assess the functioning of a family from a different ethnocultural background. There will be differences to do with value orientations and belief systems, race, family structures, and stage-specific family tasks with which the worker may be unfamiliar. There will also be differences in language and preferred modes of communication. The worker may also not know about the range of cultural defences available to members of that ethnocultural group, and what ritual activities can mediate and protect against the impacts of stresses in the group. It is therefore important that the worker is prepared for working 'in partnership' with the family by being culturally informed, and by having access to the services of a 'cultural interpreter'.

Guidelines for culturally sensitive assessments (Lau, 1991)

Life cycle issues

I will now briefly discuss life cycle issues, highlighting differences between Western European nuclear families and non-Western European traditional extended families.

Childhood and infancy

In Western European families, preparation for pregnancy is often hazardous, and pregnancy may be seen as conflicting with work or a desirable lifestyle. Families may deliberately choose not to have children.

When children are born, they develop primary bonds with biological parents, and are socialized to learn the importance of independence, individuality and assertiveness. This is reinforced by childrearing practices, e.g. sleeping alone and early weaning. Childhood stories also stress the importance of independence and working out individual-oriented solutions.

In the non-Western European extended family of Asia and Africa, young people will have been exposed to many more opportunities for sharing in childcare activities, through frequent association with the extended family. Pregnancy is often a highly desirable event, expected as an inevitable outcome of marriage.

When children are born, parenting is often shared within the wider family. As a result the child is exposed to a wider variety of parental figures and models for age and sex role identifications. Childrearing practices also reinforce notions of family inter-connectedness and group dependency, e.g. late weaning and sleeping with adults. Childhood stories not only entertain and amuse, but also educate the young child about the ideals of the group. They often stress the importance of the family and reinforce family interdependence. Recurring themes emphasize the concept of dependability and responsibility to the family and to the group (Lau, 1995; Dwivedi, 1996).

The school age child

The growing child learns from the example of family elders that he has duties towards parents and other significant adults, from whom he can expect favours. These reciprocal obligations create a system of mutual dependency that cements relationships in the family. In traditional families, people address each other not by personal names, but by kinship terms that define and locate one's position and responsibilities in the family. Duties are well defined and reinforced by socialization processes within family rituals. Thus the child learns about kinship patterns and expected relationships.

The child also learns that the important family boundary is that around the extended family. Ongoing processes within the family ensure that this boundary is maintained. Conflict resolution is not only worked out in the immediate family, but it is normal for worries to be shared in the wider family. The child also learns about family structures relevant to authority and decision making in the family, and how to access them. Thus in traditional families from Asia and Africa, blood relationships are important and age confers seniority and authority. In traditional African-Caribbean families, the household is important and may include individuals who are not related by kin, e.g. godparents or cohabitees. By virtue of longstanding association and seniority, these individuals may have authority status conferred upon them.

Children are also taught in traditional families in Asia and the Far East that one needs to be sensitive to the feelings of others, and to manage one's own feelings and aggressive impulses so they do not threaten group cohesiveness and unity. This contrasts markedly to Western ideals of self-expression, where one 'lets it all hang out'. Psychological maturity in Eastern cultures values containment of impulses and strong feelings; hence the emphasis on metaphorical and indirect communication. Religious and spiritual training in India, China and Japan focuses on the expansion of one's consciousness; identifying and accepting one's feelings, and then turning their energy to one's advantage (Dwivedi, 1996; Rimpoche, 1987).

Adolescents

The adolescent who has been exposed to socialization processes within the traditional family, will by now have internalized the rules and ego-ideals of the family system and culture, and learnt how to benefit from the resources of his family. In turn he will have learnt how to be 'dependable'. The notion of family means 'extended family', and this will have been congruent with the experience of growing up. In India, Japan, China and the Far East, most young people grow up in an extended family setting, in which 'the cultural ideal of filial loyalty and fraternal solidarity stipulates common economic and social life, common residence, ritual activities and cooking arrangements' (Dwivedi, 1996).

The traditional family will expect the young person, as part of his package of competencies, to be prepared to meet family obligations, to respect concepts of family honour, and to look after parents and younger siblings. Peer group relationships are important but must not interfere with family obligations and responsibilities. Virginity may be important to family honour, and dating by daughters may not be allowed.

In contrast, in the Western European nuclear family, the competent autonomous adolescent is expected to have a confident, separate identity. There will be increasing investment in the peer group, and he or she will be preparing to leave home. It is recognized that this is an important developmental task that needs to be negotiated and worked through, sometimes through open conflict with parents.

Traditional values in ethnic minority families are often challenged by young people, struggling within a system of dual identities, with conflict between expectations at home and expectations in the wider community of school and peer group.

Marriage and adulthood

In Western marriages a commonly accepted stage-specific task for a couple is to separate from the family of origin and to invest psychologically in the couple relationship. Individuals need to differentiate from their own families, and work out with each other issues of power and intimacy.

In the traditional non-Western family however, there are additional duties related to the wider family. The new wife in an arranged marriage within a traditional family has a different role and required obligations, with a different set of new relationships, compared to the wife in a 'love marriage'. In addition to working out her relationship with her husband, she will need to negotiate her position within the female kinship system. Particularly important will be the relationship with mother-in-law and elder sisters-in-law, all of whom will have seniority over her. Competence in the management of these new relationships will have implications on her survival and status in her new family.

The new wife in the traditional family will also be expected to support her husband's role in the patriarchal family, which will include the duty of looking after parents and younger siblings.

A suggested outline for family assessment would include the following.

What is the ethnocultural framework of the family?

The family will need to be located on the continuum between the traditional hierarchical extended family and the Western European nuclear family.

1. What belief systems influence role expectations, and define the limits of acceptable behaviour? To be effective, the worker needs access to the family's meaning systems, and to be able to determine whether or not core beliefs underlying the current problem are culturally congruent. How do the values of the group influence definitions of competence through stages in the life cycle? What are the significance of religious values and spirituality in individual and family life?
2. Practitioners commonly use normative values based on their own background and upbringing to determine what is healthy or abnormal in the assessment of individual and family functioning. They may not have access to the different cognitive orienting systems characteristic of families from a different ethnocultural group, which give rise to differences in age- and gender-based expectations of family roles. For example, the Western European worker may not share the expectation that a family has the duty to care for its aged, a common expectation in African-Caribbean families and families from Asia and Africa.
3. What family structures are relevant to authority and decision making in the family? How is the family organized to perform stage-specific tasks in the family life cycle? How are these different from norms known to the worker, and what is the impact of these differences on the work that goes on between the worker and the family?
4. What are traditional solutions used by the family and the ethnic community to resolve conflict and cope with severe stress?
5. What are the traditional networks and rituals of the family and ethnic community?
6. What are the significant stresses and losses that arise from the family's own experience in their country of origin, their adaptation to the host culture, and migration? The worker will need to be aware of the migration status of the family; what links exist between the family, the ethnic community, the host community and the emigrant community. Immigration, the loss of significant networks, the traumatic displacements that arise from the refugee experience, stresses arising out of adaptation to life in the UK, including uncertainty around refugee status and access to supportive services, can contribute to a sense of helplessness and increased risk of adversity.

Basic daily parenting tasks

Are appropriate parental tasks to do with day-to-day living being adequately performed? What is the general functioning of the adults as parents and caretakers? Are the children's developmental needs being met?

In families where the primary caretaker has suffered a relapse, it is common to find that the children have had to take on inappropriate carer roles for the ill parent. Nonetheless, there could be relative degrees of chaos and disorganization, including a lack of food in the house, and other evidence of gross neglect including inadequate clothing for the children, a fact often picked up by the school (see case example on Mira).

Family structure

What is the relevant family unit? Is there a parental couple, or is the primary caretaker the ill parent? Often where the illness has been longstanding, it is common to find that the 'well parent' has left the family home. Where there is a parental couple, the extent of marital discord and disturbance is likely to be important. The child could be drawn into the marital conflicts, and serve the purpose of distance regulation between the couple. This may then stabilize an inherently damaging family system that does not permit growth and differentiation, particularly of its children.

Where is authority located in this family? Consideration needs to be given to ethnic and cultural rules here; e.g. in traditional hierarchical extended families grandparental authority needs to be considered, as this is likely to be significant. In severely dysfunctional families skewed by a mentally ill adult, there are two common patterns. The exercise of authority could be totally inconsistent and chaotic, with a total lack of rules and structure, with confusing and unclear expectations of child behaviour. Alternatively the family system could be over-rigid and over-organized, dominated by the thinking processes of the psychotic parent who determines reality for the rest of the family.

Quality of family relationships

Here one is particularly interested in the emotional repertoire of family members. A lack of warmth, and high levels of irritability, hostility and criticism directed at the vulnerable child by the primary caretaker over a prolonged period, have been shown to have adverse outcomes. Similarly, emotional unavailability and neglect from a chronically depressed or inadequate parent lead to insecure attachments, delays in developmental tasks, and emotional and behavioural difficulties in the child.

Roles and expectations of family members

Are these appropriate within the boundaries and rules for the sexes and generations recognized by the ethnocultural group? Are there role reversals in the family, with young children expected to take on caretaking roles inappropriate to the child's age, cognitive and emotional capacities? Instead of going to school, a child may be staying at home to be with a mother with agorophobia who cannot tolerate being alone.

Ritual life of the family

It is important to know what patterned activities maintain and support structural relationships in the family. Often these activities will be prescribed by the culture, and where religious values and practices are still important, there will be religious underpinnings. They are often related to life-cycle transitions and important events; or to do with regular activities in the religious year in which participation ensures membership of the family and group, for example, fasting during Ramadan. The therapist should also be interested in rituals as a regular event of family life, e.g. dinner times together.

Rituals both in family life and in the life of the community – the storying culture of which the family is a part – are important in health maintenance and restoration to a state of well-being and competent functioning. How well placed is the therapist to activate these where they have fallen into disrepair? Or is the therapist locked into the particular vocabulary determined by their own culture of origin?

Communication

The language of communication between the worker and the family is important. Interpreters unused to the conceptual frameworks and professional language used by the team may distort or screen out important material, or at worst give the impression that effective communication has taken place between the assessment/treatment team and the family when this is not the case. Interpreters also may not be able to accurately translate ideas which are bound to the language. In Chinese, for example, ideas about feelings are often expressed in metaphorical terms, with references to the heart or the liver.

Patients whose first language is not English may feel unable to truly communicate the full extent of their distress without recourse to mother-tongue.

Case example

I had a recent case of intractable mother–daughter conflict in which the mother, a depressed Pakistani woman who had not overcome her grief at the loss of her husband through illness, was being extremely rigid and punitive with her 16-year-old daughter, who in turn was foul-mouthed and abusive to her mother, to 'get her own back'. There was a pattern of escalating conflict in which physical violence often came into play. The mother had an English vocabulary which was sufficient for day-to-day usage, but found it extremely frustrating to be unable to share her distress with me as she was unable to use English effectively. She did not have her husband around to help with bringing up the children, and her solution to coping with the uncertainties of the seductive world outside was not to let any of her children have outside friends and contacts, apart from extended family. Her daughter's response was to try to bring shame on her mother through other means, e.g. outrageous claims to behavioural excesses of various kinds, acted out in the school setting. Access to an Urdu-speaking family therapist from within my own team allowed us to keep the mother engaged, and facilitated attempts to create a therapeutic space in which issues could be re-framed in a more helpful way.

In other instances, workers' lack of familiarity with the diversity of dialect, accent and lifestyles to be found within the English-speaking world may produce some curious formulations of the predicaments faced by the people they work with. Some time ago I was asked to do an assessment in which an African-Caribbean mother, with a history of psychotic illness, was suspected by the social worker to be still delusional despite assurances from adult psychiatric staff to the contrary. The social worker (UK White) said the mother was still wiping her 4-year-old daughter's bottom, and talking about 'cocks' running about the house, so was possibly overly involved sexually with her daughter. When I saw the mother, she had an extremely heavy Jamaican accent, and tended to speak loudly in an agitated manner. Her formal mental state, however, was intact. Her primary concern was to be rehoused and she showed me correspondence from her surveyors documenting the extent of damp, infestation etc, in her house. She was worried about the cockroaches running around the place and spent time trying to catch them. At this interview her little girl asked to go to the toilet, and the mother expressed concern that the child had still not learnt to clean herself properly. When the child emerged from the toilet I asked to see the child's bottom. The child had not wiped herself and there was faecal material around her anal opening. I felt that the child needed toilet training and better hygiene, rather than being a child in need of protection from possible sexual abuse.

With severely disturbed families, attention must be paid to the extent of distortion of communication, and mystification. Are communications clear and direct, or intrusive and 'mind-invasive'? Do conversations lead anywhere? The following case illustrates the parent's inability to focus on issues in discussions with her son, who she felt totally dominated her. The quality of the conversation between the two of them showed strange patterns, and it was an effort for the therapist to follow the thread of conversation.

Case example

Sandra, who lived by herself with her 9-year-old son David, had just been discharged from psychiatric hospital following an admission with a diagnosis of paranoid schizophrenia. The referring adult psychiatrist was concerned about her capacity to maintain appropriate boundaries with her son. At the age of 9 years, she was still wiping his bottom.

I saw Sandra with David. At the time she was no longer suffering from acute symptoms, and had stabilized on medication. The main concern, she said, was that David kept arguing with her and trying to dominate her. This lady's sense of reality had been quite tenuous, as she was often subject to taking action on her child's behalf under the influence of auditory hallucinations. A question about what school this boy attended was responded to as follows:

David: 'Uh, what school is it Mum?'
Sandra: 'He goes to School A. It used to be School B, but I never felt comfortable there. Neither did David. Then my voices said I should take him away'.
Dr Lau: 'How did you feel about leaving your friends at School B?'
David: 'I used to miss them but I made new friends'.
Sandra: 'It's much better at School A'.

The following exchange took place in response to my question to David about how he got on with his Mum.

David: 'My Mum tells lies about me. She says she'll put me in a home'.
Dr Lau: 'What kinds of lies?'
David: 'She says I haven't tidied my room when I have. She gets angry'.
Sandra: 'You didn't tidy your room. You don't help me when I want you to go with me to the supermarket. Don't I love you? Don't I do things for you?'
David: 'What things did you do for me?'

Sandra: 'Didn't I buy those colouring pens you wanted?'
David: 'But they weren't the ones I wanted! I wanted [describes type and brand].
          That's what all my friends have'.
Sandra: 'The ones I got were much better'.
David: 'I want to go home now. I want to take a taxi home'.
Sandra: 'The 158 bus will take us home door to door'.
David: 'No, I'm not going home by bus, I want a taxi!'

Sandra admitted that her conversations with her son were like her conversations with herself. They never came to a clear conclusion, but drifted into mindless space.

Belief system

What is the cognitive orienting structure of the family? Is this congruent with the ethnocultural context? Or do the distortions arise from the impaired mental functioning of the sick parent, e.g. 'the educational system is dominated by evil ideas'? Where the delusional system involves one or more of the children, then there is a direct risk to the child's safety.

Behaviour controls

Of particular concern is the finding of parental violence, or potential threats against the children; severe behavioural disturbance, e.g. drugs, alcohol; self-destructive acts, repeated suicide attempts. It is important to find out what has happened to the exercise of authority in the traditional extended family, which would normally serve the function of providing a source for mediating family conflict, as well as containing and restraining extreme behavioural disturbance in any one family member.

Assessment of the parent

It is important to take a longitudinal developmental history, focusing on the individual's history of relationships, and also on all past and current stresses to which the individual is vulnerable. In taking a psychiatric history one also looks at the severity and chronicity of the condition. We know that severity and chronicity of parental illness has more impact on a child's development than a one-off episode with periods of good functioning in between. How stable is the parent's mental state, if in a stage of remission? What is the likelihood of further relapses? The history of previous involvement with mental health services, including the degree of cooperation with treatment, is important in determining future patterns of compliance with a treatment programme.

The general functioning of the parent requires assessment, as does the extent to which his or her mental health impairment has affected the parenting role and tasks. A depressed mother is vulnerable to being overwhelmed by uncontrollable affective states or urges. The illness process interferes with her capacity to be a consistent and sensitive attachment figure for her child (Hill, 1996). She is often emotionally unavailable, with a limited emotional range, unable to respond to the verbal or nonverbal cues from the child. These patients commonly describe feelings of helplessness when confronted by the normal needs and demands of the child or young infant. They may ascribe inappropriate intentions to their child's behaviour, or fail to recognize the child as having separate needs from herself. Often adequate boundaries are not maintained.

A mother I once saw treated her 10-year-old daughter almost as an older confidante, and talked to her in detail about her problems with men friends. The child became very confused about her role, and boundaries. There were conflicting messages as to whether she was a dependent child, who took orders from her mother; or was she in fact her mother's mother, who had to look after a mother incapable of looking after herself. If the latter was the case, then by implication she did not have to take mother's authority demands that seriously.

Where a good supportive personal network is not available, the sick parent often induces the child into a caretaking role. The incompatibility of that role with the child's needs as a dependent young person for an external source of adult authority in order that the child may have a secure internalized sense of self, often leads to behavioural difficulties seen as 'conflicts with authority'.

I am sometimes also asked to assess the partners of mentally ill adults who are considered dangerous, for example with a diagnosis of paranoid schizophrenia and an established pattern of violent behaviour. The partners are usually mothers, with dependent children. The issue that needs to be considered is often the capacity of the mother to protect the children from damaging contact with the abusive parent.

Case example

A recent case was one in which the mother, a young woman of African-Caribbean background, felt unable for a long time to resist pressure from her husband's relatives to take her husband back after his numerous discharges from hospital. She felt a strong sense of duty to continue to care for her husband. The father had a diagnosis of paranoid schizophrenia, and at the point of referral of his son to me for assessment, was in a secure hospital setting for beating up his guards. In the recent past he had repeatedly assaulted his wife when he suffered paranoid relapses, following lack of compliance with medication. After a series of particularly severe attacks, the mother finally called the police, and now lived in fear of retribution from her husband for 'putting him away'.

The referred patient was aged 13 years. Social Services asked for an assessment to determine whether he should be removed from the care of his mother, who had in the past made 'no attempts to protect the boy from damaging contact with his father'. As a result, he experienced difficulties in school related to lack of concentration and poor school attendance, was extremely behind in his work and found it difficult to catch up. This in turn had a negative impact on his motivation to continue going to school, which he saw as a place where he received continual criticism for inadequate school achievement. He had traumatic memories of witnessing attacks on his mother by his father when the father was under the influence of voices, who told him his wife was unfaithful. At the same time however, he also had good memories of his father, who, when well and in control, had spent time doing things with his son. He remembered his father as being well for long periods, though about once a year over the past few years his father would become ill and then his behaviour would be violent and bizarre. He was sorry for his father, he said, because it was not really his father who beat his mother up, it was father's illness. At the same time he remembered things his father would say that would upset him, including the idea that he was 'just like him' and would eventually become mad like him. The boy told me he did not want to leave his mother, and would run away back home to her if attempts were made to remove him. He was sure that his mother meant what she had told him, i.e. that she was determined not to let his father return, as she now believed the chances of the father maintaining a stable mental state were poor. He told me he agreed with his mother's decision.

I found the mother and son to have a close and warm relationship, in which the boy was described as extremely helpful at home and not a discipline problem in any way. School was the main issue, and the boy would find ways of waking up late and going in late. The mother did not get on with her allocated social worker. Communications with Social Services were erratic, with a lack of trust on both sides. Social Services saw her as unreliable and inconsistent, putting her son at risk by continuing to live with a dangerous man. My assessment of the situation was that the boy should be supported in staying at home with his mother, and helped to sort out issues around school attendance and school competence. I also made attempts to get him to talk about his fears and worries around his father, but he resolutely refused to discuss these matters.

Eventually however, the mother used resources from her church and religious faith to become more assertive of her rights and needs. She was then able to be clearer as well as firmer with her expectations of her son and help him with his problematic school attendance.

An earlier professional network meeting about this family raised the issue of conflicting professional views, which arose from different frames of reference. The adult psychiatrist said her patient's mental state was now stable, and it was important to his self-esteem to retain his parental role and status as otherwise he faced a bleak and barren future. The loss of his child would have catastrophic consequences and hinder his long-term rehabilitation (Hill, 1996). It was therefore unnecessary to maintain a stance that denied this father access to his child, even if the child did not wish it; the child should be persuaded that contact with their father would be in their best interests. The child psychiatrist felt, however, that there was an overwhelming imperative to protect the child who had already suffered 'significant harm', and described being traumatized by exposure to the father's episodic violence. The social worker said there was a long-term, recurrent pattern of relapses due to the father's inconsistent compliance with medication.

It was also interesting the way the 'black perspective' operated to produce differences of professional opinion in this case. The allocated social worker (African-Caribbean) said that because this was a black boy we were dealing with, he had special needs and should be removed from home for his own good and placed in a special school for black children where he could receive more intensive educational therapy. This would however mean leaving home and the lad would have none of it. Both the boy and his mother preferred that he should stay at home and work towards a better school adjustment. The differences in views however led to tensions in the relationship between the social worker and the mother.

Assessment of the child

The interview and observations of the child need to be tailored to the child's age, level of understanding and cultural context. Often drawings, toys and a doll's house are used to help younger children express themselves. We are interested in assessing the child's state of development, including physical, cognitive and psychological parameters. Is the child achieving key tasks of social and emotional development appropriate to its age? Children of depressed mothers generally show poor cognitive and speech development, with long-term effects, resulting from lack of appropriate stimulation (Puckering, 1989). There are areas of psychological deficits stemming from poor attachment experiences. The young child may show disturbed patterns of attachment, ranging from 'insecure avoidant' and 'insecure ambivalent' to 'disorganized' (Ainsworth et al., 1978).

Areas of assessment include:

- physical development, including ill-health;
- cognitive development;
- emotional development;
- the child's current behaviour at home and school;
- mental processes, including defences against anxiety;
- relationships within the family, with parents, siblings and significant others in the extended family.

We usually request the school to provide information regarding the child's competence at school tasks, and his relationships with peers and teachers.

Where there is a history of childhood disturbance, it is important to look at the age of onset, persistence and stability of the problem.

It is particularly important to look at the following:

1. The child's understanding of the parent's illness.
2. The extent to which the child has been exposed to traumatic incidents (e.g. cruelty, sexual assault, violence directed at family members, traumatic hospitalization of parent).
3. The child's fears and fantasies. Does the child feel responsible for the ill parent? Does the child need to protect the parent by staying home from school? What is the level of confusion when confronted with the parent's delusions, hallucinations, bizarre and fragmented thoughts? How does the child cope with guilt over his/her wish for removal of the disturbed parent?
4. Is the child socially isolated and bullied or stigmatized by having a parent who is mentally ill?
5. What is the child's total experience of the ill parent? Is the parental illness chronic and severe? Or were there periods of adequate functioning punctuated by crises due

to parental breakdown? What compensatory measures were employed by the child in order to cope? Is the child the target of the parent's paranoid projections?

Not all children with mentally-ill parents suffer significant harm. Children who have been anxious prior to parental illness are more likely to suffer from post-traumatic stress disorders. Children who have been more 'involved' in the parental illness are more likely to have long-term impairment of relationships and poor outcomes. Resilient children are those who have been able to get used to the recurrent stresses, and devote their energies to their school and peer group (Anthony, 1986).

The time to worry is when children present with evidence of impaired functioning. In my experience one of the commonest is school failure – either from an inability to concentrate in a learning situation, or arising from the need to stay at home in order to look after the sick parent. The child will often be too preoccupied by their worries about things going on at home to be able to get on with school-based tasks. These children are often emotionally inhibited and constricted, often fiercely loyal to the sick parent and unwilling to be parted from them.

Children may also be at risk from the lengthy deliberations of well-meaning professionals who allow children to wait for long periods of time in temporary placements. This may have to do with assessing the feasibility of rehabilitation to the ill parent; or in waiting for legal proceedings to take place; or to secure the 'correct' adoptive placement. There are also cases in which a high staff turnover, combined with use of temporary (agency) staff, has led to lack of continuity in planning and service provision, including case allocation. For younger children in particular, the impact of repeated separations from attachment figures at a vulnerable period in the child's life can be particularly damaging. This predisposes to an inability to form trusting relationships, with attendant emotional and behavioural disturbances with long-term effects, including the development of severe antisocial personality disorders in adulthood (Zeitlin, 1986; Hall, 1996).

Case example

A referral was made by the headteacher of a primary school on two children, Mira aged 8 years, and her brother Adil, aged 5 years. We were told the mother was at the time an inpatient in the local psychiatric hospital. There was also a baby of 7 months. The children were being cared for by their stepfather and grandmother. The school was concerned about the impact of numerous allegations made by the mother directed at Mira, before she went into hospital. This included accusations that Mira had sexually abused her mother. The school noted Mira appeared to be 'missing her mother and was seeking one of the school secretaries out on a daily basis in order to talk about her worries. It would take a long time to coax her back to class. Her schoolwork was suffering as she seeks attention in class also, or she sits and broods'. The school requested support in order to help the child 'balance what she has seen and heard, and to help make sense of the present situation'.

This case was regarded by our intake team as urgent and was immediately allocated. At the family meeting which was held shortly afterwards, it was clear to us that the mother, Mrs Ahmad, who was then on leave from the inpatient unit, was still quite unwell. She was labile, loud and aggressive, and in front of both young children made numerous accusations that not only was her husband unfaithful, but that he had sexually abused Mira. She got ill and had to be admitted into hospital, she said, because her husband spends the whole day outside the home, and she knows he is sexually abusing Mira because Mira has diarrhoea. Mira also 'looks' like she has been abused; in fact her husband abuses her while she is asleep. She said she told the social worker a few months ago but this was not investigated. She did not pursue the matter for fear that the children might be removed from her. It was likely that the children were abused while she was in hospital. Father denied these allegations. He loved her, he said, but she had ruined his life with her illness, and he had not known about her illness when he married her. Yes, it was an arranged marriage, he said. He had lied at the ward meeting the day before and said Mrs Ahmad was improving when actually she was not. This resulted in the decision, which he now regretted, of her being on leave from the Unit for 2 weeks. (About 2 weeks ago she had had to be sectioned under the Mental Health Act in order to enable her to receive treatment.)

We then saw Mira on her own. She had been very quiet and subdued in the earlier meeting, and had tried to distract herself with the toys in the room. She was tearful and distressed after her parents left the room, and said she did not like it when her parents argued. She wanted her Mummy at home because Mummy looks after her and helps her with her homework. We asked Mira what she thought about what her mother said her father (actually her stepfather) had done to her. Mira said many of the arguments between her parents were over Mummy saying Daddy was going out to have sex with girls. She said she did not know what 'sex' was. We then introduced the anatomically explicit dolls, and established the names she used for various genitalia. She denied inappropriate touching of these areas by her father. She said however that Mummy keeps asking her if Daddy had done dirty things to her. In the end she had to say he had done it, otherwise Mummy would keep going on about it. She did not know what else to do, she said, and then became very upset. She said her mother had not touched her in a dirty way, but again became quite upset. She said her brother had told lies, about how she had touched her mother's genitals when her mother was asleep. Her brother had also once told her one of father's friends had touched him in the genital area and that he did not like it. She did not want us to tell her mother what she had said, as her mother would only tell her off. We felt however, that we had to confront the issues with Mrs Ahmad.

The rest of the family was invited back in and we went over what Mira had told us. Mrs Ahmad then became very angry. She said Mira was too scared to tell the truth, and in any case we were not qualified to diagnose child sexual abuse. She continued to accuse her husband of having affairs, and appeared labile and possibly deluded. She terminated the interview abruptly and announced she was taking her family home.

Our impressions from the meeting were that the mother was still unwell, with manic and paranoid symptoms. We also felt the children, especially Mira, were at risk of emotional abuse and possibly neglect. There was on file a history of concerns from the school and others, including the health visitor, that the children were sometimes not fed properly, e.g. milk being given to the baby that was too hot; the children were often inappropriately dressed for school; and it was also unclear whether there was sexual abuse going on and who might be involved.

The case was reported to the duty social worker at the relevant children and families team in the local authority. A few days later we heard that a social worker had been around to the house and found Mrs Ahmad to be 'reasonably stable and there was no apparent cause for concern'. It turned out our own concerns, expressed over the phone, had been passed down the line to various people and we suspected that specific enquiries had not been made. We decided our concerns and findings had to be distributed in written form to the various parties, and a strategy meeting convened.

This eventually took the form of a Section 117 meeting on the ward, and the meeting was attended by the consultant psychiatrist in charge of the Unit, a psychiatrist from our team, the approved social worker (for the mother), a social worker from the children and families team, the senior social worker from the team, the community psychiatric nurse who had been seeing the mother in the community, the health visitor, and the headteacher for the children. The meeting was extremely useful in resolving differences of view in the professional network, and led to an agreed strategy for action. At this meeting, both the adult and the child psychiatrists were united in asserting their views on Mrs Ahmad's continuing fragility, and the extremely high likelihood of relapse of her condition. The family had come from a different borough, with a history of physical abuse by the mother. There had been a previous lengthy child abuse investigation prompted by Mrs Ahmad's allegations that Mira was evil, and had sexually abused her through the power of her mind. As there had been no positive findings, the social workers had decided that was not an area they were going to look at in the initial home visit. It was felt they had an inadequate understanding of the chronic relapsing nature of Mrs Ahmad's illness.

The mental health services had found her to be difficult to engage, lacking insight into her condition, and not compliant with medication. The health visitor reported ongoing concerns about Mrs Ahmad's management of the baby, who appeared to have a 'frozen' attitude. At one point, she was scared for her own safety when threatened by Mrs Ahmad and had to leave the house; this was just prior to Mrs Ahmad's admission to hospital under the Mental Health Act. Also the husband had now left the family.

Mrs Ahmad's social worker also noted that the mother had overfed and shaken the baby in her presence. Mrs Ahmad was resistant to the need to engage with other professionals, and said her main need was for housing and finances. In fact she wanted to be rehoused in another borough in order to be closer to her own family. The school expressed concern about the care being given to the baby and the children by the mother, and also Mira's needy and depressed state in school. She was underachieving, with a delay of 3 years. It was only after the headteacher phoned the previous school that she found out that the mother had a previous history of mental illness.

There was a vast amount of delusional sexual material expressed by the mother, to which the children had been exposed on an ongoing basis. We felt that the mother's delusional symptoms were persisting, even though on the surface she might be coping with the daily demands of housework and childcare. The mother was now caring for the children on her own without support from family or friends. The family had also moved around a great deal; this was the fourth borough, and mother wanted to move again.

The senior social worker assured the meeting that this would be a priority case for allocation. They would then do a comprehensive assessment, including the child protection issues.

Since that meeting there has been intense monitoring of the family, and Mrs Ahmad indicated she would be willing to meet with us again.

Recommendations to managers of services

1. A strategy meeting with the professional network needs to be convened in all cases where children of parents with mental health problems are at risk.
   a) All relevant information needs to be shared amongst all the interested parties, in order that there is an agreed view taken about any risk to the child. Child protection procedures need to be activated if this is relevant, including allocation of the case to a social worker with statutory responsibilities.
   b) Ensure the ill parent's treatment needs are being met.
   c) Plan for direct psychotherapeutic work with the affected child or young person. This should include discussion of the child's ambivalence towards the ill parent. The therapist provides a space in which the child can openly discuss his fears and fantasies with a 'safe' adult, and be confronted by the demands of reality. The sessions with the child are aimed at correcting incongruencies of affect and communication, and diminishing magical and superstitious beliefs imposed by a psychotic parent.
2. Family work to consolidate support structures, and to enhance competence and reality testing. Mobilize strengths, e.g. work on reducing high levels of expressed emotion (hostility, criticism) with families with a schizophrenic member.

Case example

This is a piece of clinical work currently in progress.

Jonathan is a 6-year-old boy whose mother, Claire, aged 22 years, has suffered from paranoid schizophrenia for at least 5 years, with a history of four acute admissions to hospital. His mother has lived with a lesbian partner for a considerable period. This woman, Jill, has undertaken the majority of parenting tasks with respect to Jonathan, including meal preparation, housework and childcare. Sometimes Jonathan's mother would read to him at bedtime. Two weeks prior to our first meeting with Jonathan, his mother was again admitted to hospital under a hospital section. This time the stresses of coping with her sick partner were too much for Jill, and the boy was placed rather precipitously with his maternal grandparents. Jonathan has had no contact with his own father since he was 1 year old, and the father died 6 months ago.

Three years ago Jonathan had been referred by the paediatric registrar for 'severe auto-destructive disturbances including headbanging and self-biting'. At that time he had been living with foster parents for 6 months, and his mother was in psychiatric hospital for a 3-month period. By the time they were seen, Jonathan was back home with his mother and her partner. The family were referred to a parenting group but failed to take up the offer.

Recent concern had been expressed from the school as Jonathan was behaving strangely, and talking about vampires and witches as if they were real. Once he put his hands around a boy's neck. The grandparents told us he was saying strange things like pressing a particular button would produce a deadly ball of fire; or he wanted to cut or hurt himself to be like his mother. With his mother, he was often clingy and protective.

Jill told us that it had been really scary for her in recent weeks. Claire would come crying into the bathroom while Jill was having a bath, and say her voices wanted her to drown Jill in the bath. In the past Jill had covered up for Claire when she had refused to take her medication, so that the community psychiatric nurse would not be alarmed. She insisted, however, that both she and Claire tried to ensure that Jonathan did not know about his mother's delusions and voices, and had not been exposed directly to them: 'Claire would tell me instead of telling him.'

In the course of an individual interview with Jonathan we realized that Jill was quite mistaken, and Jonathan had in fact been exposed to a lot of his mother's delusional material. Jonathan was a bright and articulate boy, who was missing Jill more than he missed his mother. In the early part of the session he was very restless and talked incessantly. When asked why he thought his mother was in hospital, he said it was because she had headaches. She also used to kick and punch the wall, and also hits and slaps herself, he said. She tells him she loves him. At other times she says she is a vampire and he did not like it when she said that. He would try to go to his room 'until she stops saying that'. We asked if Jill would help him when he was frightened, and he said sometimes Jill took him off to her parents' house.

Jonathan drew pictures of 'friendly dinosaurs' with sharp teeth that he said he needed to have around him as they stopped the vampires from getting to him. His mother had told him the ghosts and vampires were real, he said; in fact they could go anywhere, including the interview room.

We felt Jonathan came across as an extremely anxious child, who had been traumatized by being repeatedly exposed to his mother's psychotic fantasies. The separation from Jill, who had been his primary caretaker, had been abrupt and he did not have a chance to make any sense of it. It was important for this boy to be seen on an individual basis, in order to have space to explore concerns about his mother, but also to support the demands of reality testing.

Jonathan brought a few of his own dinosaur toys with him to the first individual session. One was a special toy, whom Jonathan described as his special friend, who came to life at night and protected him: 'He scares off the other monsters.' When the therapist attempted to challenge this, he became quite upset and insisted it was real. We felt this toy had characteristics of a transitional object for Jonathan, and helped him negotiate the boundary between reality and fantasy in an ego-supportive way. A few days later his grandmother telephoned to tell us the boy had been upset following the session, and had laid down on the floor and asked her to hit and kick him, 'just like Mummy'.

In subsequent sessions Jonathan continued to bring his dinosaur, Barnaby, but was then able to say all dinosaurs were dead and lived in the past. He was no longer scared of them as they were all dead. He told the therapist he had 'helped make the scary monsters go'. At the same time he talked less about his mother, and would build houses in which mother was absent. He was rather anxious about leaving sessions, and wanted to be sure the therapist preserved an image of him, as well as space for him for following sessions. He also revisited themes of locking bad people away. (His mother was still in hospital.) It was difficult to talk about his mother directly, and he admitted 'my head goes wrong when I think about Mum', and that talking about her made him have bad dreams about alligators.

Around this time there was a Care Programme Approach meeting on the psychiatric ward that we attended, in which it came to light that Claire had had thoughts of harming Jonathan. We therefore recommended that for the time being, she should not have unsupervised access to him. The plan is that individual work with Jonathan should continue, and we would be contributing to multi-agency discussions on his long-term placement needs. Jonathan needs to have his own allocated social worker, and formal arrangements need to be in place around his placement with his grandparents, which at the moment is strictly on an informal and voluntary basis. Jonathan is obviously showing us that his experiences of his mother are difficult to process at this time, and in fact he is not able to talk to his therapist about her without worrying that it will produce bad dreams. A few days ago we heard from the ward that Claire is asking to see Jonathan. From an adult treatment perspective this would help Claire in her rehabilitation as it activates her expectations of resuming normal roles, i.e. that of parenting. We feel however that access to his mother at this time may not be in Jonathan's best interests.

Recommendations to purchasers of services (health and social care)

Purchasers need to redress the current splits in service delivery, in which services for adult mental health, and child and adolescent mental health services are often separate, with a gulf between staff training and practice in the respective service areas. Service specifications for mental health services must include screening and identification of the mental health needs of dependent children in a family where the parent is mentally ill. Similarly the splits of responsibility inherent in the different roles of the social workers in children and families teams, and community mental health teams (CMHT), mean that the needs of the family are often not addressed.

Acknowledgements

I wish to acknowledge the contributions of the following: Dr Mark Woodgate, Registrar in Child Psychiatry, for his individual work with 'Jonathan', Dr Sam Marriott, Staff Grade Psychiatrist, for her work with 'Mrs Ahmad and family and Ms Shila Khan, Family Therapist, for her work with the Pakistani Urdu speaking family.

The above are members of the staff team at Redbridge Child and Family Consultation Centre, Ilford, Essex.

The user's perspective: the experience of being a parent with a mental health problem

Nigel Phillips and Richard Hugman

Surveys of literature indicate that existing research on parents with psychiatric disorders showed amongst other things that there were likely to be higher rates of family discord and persistent emotional disorders in both the partner and the children of the ill person (Rutter and Quinton, 1984).

Our own previous experience as social workers in generic teams in the 1980s suggested that families where one parent had a serious mental health problem tended in some cases to give rise to concerns about the welfare or safety of the children. Fisher *et al.* (1984) noted that social work practice in area teams tended to emphasize the needs of children, with parents' needs being seen as secondary or else ignored. Also they surveyed social workers rather than service users. No attempt appears in the research literature to ask parents how they coped with bringing up children whilst themselves suffering from a mental illness, and what effect it had on the parent–child relationship. This chapter reports on a small-scale in-depth qualitative study, undertaken to explore these questions and in order to find out how parents with a mental health problem experienced the services that were meant to be available to them and what, if any, views they had about possible improvements in those services.

The study looks at the perceptions of 24 people in four different service settings in an industrial city in the north of England. Sixteen of the interviewees were women whilst eight of them were men. All were self-selected volunteers who had agreed to meet with one of us following an introductory talk at each of the service centres. The numbers of interviewees in the different settings is shown in Table 10.1.

The key common factors are that all of the interviewees had experience of mental health problems and of being parents. All had used professional services, including social work (in which we had a particular interest given our own professional work backgrounds). The interviews, which took place between May 1991 and May 1992, were based on a short list of open-ended questions which asked about the person's experience of mental illness, their experience of being a parent, their perception of links between the two, and their responses to the professional services they had

Table 10.1 Location of service users interviewed

Location	Women	Men	Total
SSD day centre	3	2	5
Voluntary organization drop-in	5	4	9
DHA day hospital	3	2	5
Resource centre*	5	0	5
Total	16	8	24

*Multi-disciplinary, jointly run by SSD and DHA.

received. The interviews were tape-recorded (with the explicit permission of each person). The transcriptions were then analysed using the 'induction' approach described by Burgess (1984), which involves a qualitative analysis of responses in order to derive analytic themes. It is these thematic ideas, expressed so far as possible in the respondent's own words which served to structure our reporting of the research.

It is important to note that the interviews were conducted with parents and that, in this study, the absence of children's views was intentional. We are obviously aware that the voice of children has, with the exception of researchers such as Webster (1992), seldom been heard in the sort of situations of which our respondents are but a small sample. Our aim, however, was to talk to parents and find out what their experience had been. Whether or not the child's perspective would reveal differences or similarities between the two perspectives must await further research in the area.

Effects on the parenting experience

Although we did not incorporate a specific question about diagnosis, it became clear that our respondents had all suffered from a severe mental disorder (schizophrenia, manic depressive illness or postnatal depression invariably featured in the accounts they gave us) which had had a profound impact on their family life and in particular on their ability to be a successful parent. Crucial to our understanding is the notion of loss of parental role, or 'missed parenting', which varied from an inability to respond to their children's routine needs to temporary or permanent separation (because of divorce, adoption and so on). In particular we recognized certain changes in parental responsibility which arose not only from their own mental health problems, but also out of a range of normative expectations as to how parents should behave. We will now go on to explore these losses and changes in more detail.

Loss of existing parental role

For our respondents, this included the energy needed for everyday activities, the loss of which figured as a significant diminution of their abilities as parents, particularly of young children. This is illustrated by one mother who told us:

'We go to the playgroup down there, which is about five minutes walk away, but when I was ill I couldn't even walk down there by myself. I had to ring a friend up to take her . . .'

A father who was recovering from a severe mental illness and was separated from his wife and small son describes the activities he would like to pursue with him on regular access visits:

'He wants to be occupied in (activities) like swimming or football (. . .) but I find with the medication slowing me down so much I just don't have the capacity to keep going, whereas before I could just keep going all day.'

In total, six of our interviewees mentioned reduced levels of energy and motivation in dealing with the demands of their children. A different order of loss of parental role is brought about by separation as a result of the parent being admitted to a psychiatric hospital, a theme explored by over 50 per cent of our respondents. While visits in some cases mitigated the loss and separation for parent and child, the experience was not always a helpful one, as the following example illustrates:

'(My wife) did bring the children up twice when I had my first breakdown. There were all the other patients saying 'What are you bringing kids up here for?'

Hospital visits by no means constitute reassurance that a parent would remain a presence in the child's life, with this example of the fear of the mother's re-admission following discharge home expressed by the child aged 5 years:

'She would come to me and cry, she didn't want to go to school. She clung on my coat and cried. She thought I would be taken away again'.

As well as the breakdown of direct care caused by the parent's admission to hospital, and the putting at risk of the child's expectation that the parent will always be there for them, another form of loss was described by a number of our respondents, that of authority in the family. This would appear to be brought about by the parent's disappearance from the child's life at the time of hospital admission, or as a consequence of changes in his or her behaviour emanating from their mental illness. One respondent who had attempted to bring up four children largely on her own describes the difficulties of exerting parental authority:

'I think they've got an easy life really because (when) I am poorly I tend to give in more than be as firm as what I should be.'

The dilemma involved in showing love and affection on the one side whilst displaying authority and consistency on the other, was particularly hard for these parents struggling with their own mental health problems. Given that a majority of our sample were (or had been) single parents, a loss of parental authority was likely to have profound consequences for the future stability of the family.

A different anxiety mentioned by three of our respondents was that produced largely by the stigma associated with having a mental illness, and the awareness that the demeaning status associated with that stigma can all too easily be absorbed even by one's children, and repeated back to the parent at times of family stress. One mother described how her older children had picked up this currency of stigma and stereotyping and used it to undermine her authority in the family thus:

'The kids used to say "you're always poorly, you're always sick, you're mental, you are".'

The notion of the missed (or altered) experience of parenting takes on a deeper meaning of loss where a respondent has given up parenting altogether when particular stresses have built up either due to a mental health crisis or to circumstances in the family, or both. These events correlate with the positive support role played by a range of alternative carers, usually from within the extended family itself. The majority of such arrangements emerged from the children's' own grandparents, with the respondent's own family and that of his/her partner's family being about equally represented as the temporary carers amongst our respondents. However where extended family were unable to help, or where there was a long-running decline in the mental health of the parent, or a decline in their ability to adequately play a parenting role, there was a resort to more formal care arrangements such as the children being received into the care of the local authority. We encountered five such situations amongst our respondents. This mother is a typical example:

'(My daughter) was put in care. My husband put her in care: he was working and he couldn't afford to have the time off work (. . .). When I first got took into hospital, I wasn't able to think at all . . .'

Ultimately long-term or repeated episodes of mental ill-health led in some cases to the interviewee's right to parent her/his children at all being called into question. In such situations the now ex-partner may decide to pursue legal steps to assume custody of the children. In one example a mother who had been in hospital for some time told us:

'The court welfare officer was asking questions about why I felt I should have custody of the children (. . .) which was difficult because I never saw them at that time. Actually they paid more attention to their dad. They seemed to feel that I had walked out and left them . . .'

A 'double oppression' can be seen in the lives of these parents: not only do they have serious mental health problems but they also were now faced with being formally denied any future care of their children. Such individuals were seldom sufficiently empowered to take legal redress, whether against an ex-partner, or against a local authority taking care proceedings. These particular parents' stories are made poignant by virtue of being caught between concentrating on their own needs and thereby underwriting a professional view of themselves as inadequate parents, or desperately pursuing what seems to be a fast-disappearing parenting role. One woman who was suffering a severe postnatal depression, and was living with a violent partner at the time of the child's birth, told us:

> 'They told me when my son was about 8 weeks old that I had to choose between my husband and my child, which was a terrible experience, and I chose my child . . .'

While these comments fairly represent the majority of our respondents, our survey does not thankfully present a universal catalogue of losses, and it is appropriate to move on briefly to consider some of the positive role changes and coping strategies which our interviewees described.

Becoming a parent

A general distinction was noted between those people who had become parents after having mental health problems, and those whose mental ill-health followed having a child. Our evidence suggests that whilst the latter group were more likely to face disruption in relationships with their children, the former group (eight of our sample told us they had a pre-existing mental health problem before they had any children) were in some cases able to consider whether becoming a parent was the right thing in the circumstances. The challenge of assuming new roles through becoming parents is one that most of our interviewees mentioned. In the main our respondents, albeit with the benefit of hindsight, felt they had made the right decision to start families. Perhaps acquisition of the parental role may not only fulfil deeper emotional needs, but may actually confer a degree of normative status upon individuals whose lives up to that point have been systematically devalued through having a mental illness. One couple, who were both mental health service users, explained their decision about becoming parents in this way:

> 'Well, we knew it was going to be difficult, (but) we'd been in a relationship for a long time, about 3 years, and it was pretty stable, and so we decided to have (our child).'

The experience of many of these parents has tended towards added concern over their children's future as a result both of immersion in the parent's mental illness, and what some saw as the danger of 'passing it on to the child', albeit in a way that the parent themselves didn't entirely understand. One mother explained it to us like this:

> 'I just wonder if she can remember it (episodes of the mother's mental illness), or if it will affect her, or is she going to go like me? (. . .) It has affected me that way as I don't want her to grow up like me, I want her to be happy . . .'

A second example of a successful assumption of new roles emerges from evidence that some of our respondent's second marriages appeared to be happier and more stable than first ones, particularly if the earlier relationship (and children from it) came at a time which coincided with a mental health breakdown. One father, whose previous partner had taken out an injunction to prevent him seeing her and their child at the end of a marriage beset by his mental health problems, was able to describe his present situation thus:

'I've got married again and got two stepchildren. They know I've been mentally ill but they don't make a big thing of it. They don't talk behind my back and they respect me within reason (. . .). My wife, when I first met her and told her about it, she wouldn't believe it, she thought I was having her on.'

Moving on to a second and possibly more successful marriage, may also bring with it the likelihood of a step-parenting relationship, thereby bringing further stresses for the new family. On being asked how the subject of mental illness is treated in the family, the same stepfather said:

'We very rarely talk about it in front of the children, because I think a lot of the things which I've experienced like hallucinations are scary, and would make them feel differently towards me . . .'

Role reversal

Evidence has emerged from earlier research (Webster, 1992) that the children of parents with mental health problems may themselves take on key aspects of caring for their parent(s). Our own research suggests a subtle variety of role change in parent–child interactions which are in certain ways different from those seen to operate for children of parents suffering from chronic physical disabilities (Barnardos, 1992). The differences can be summarized thus:

1. whilst the demands of physical caring may be less onerous, the demand for emotional support will predominate, with all the attendant difficulties for a child in responding to such requests.
2. mental illness is likely to be spasmodic, fluctuating in its occurrence or degree of seriousness and often unpredictable. For the child who lacks an understanding of these facts, or is of an age at which he or she is unable to fully appreciate them, the care that he or she can give is likely to spontaneously reflect, or even anticipate, the parent's emotional state.

One of our respondents talked about the role performed by her pre-teenage son. From this and other interviews we obtained a strong sense not only of household tasks being taken over but also of emotional support being given in ways that anticipate, or seek to prevent, parental breakdown:

'He looked after me. If I was doing something, he'd say "no, I'll do that" (. . .) there's certain things you do and he can tell (from) the way I act that I'm getting poorly, because he'll say "are you getting poorly again?" and that brings you round . . .'

Ultimately the mother whom we earlier noted as expressing concern about how her child would grow up describes the support she is getting from her own child as follows:

'I was very worried, I used to sit crying and stuff, and it was just like a role reversal, she used to come and put her arms around me and fetch me books and things. I used to think, well, how is it going to affect her?'

Another respondent who was also a single parent told us of times when the only thing which stopped her from harming herself (an aspect of her longstanding mental health problem) was the presence of her 2-year-old, who would comfort and show affection to her mother.

'Sometimes when she knows that I'm upset, she'll come up to me, she'll start cuddling me or make me laugh (. . .) it's as though she's doing it deliberately, saying "come on, mum, cheer up . . ."'

Coping strategies

There were in fact a whole range of other informal strategies adopted by our respondents in facing a fluctuating mental health problem. These ranged from the development of preventative routines in the home through to attempts to confront the impact of past abuses in the life of the adult on her present ability to parent successfully. A routine strategy was stressed by one woman as follows:

'If you have a mental health need, you make sure the children are safe because you're on guard all the time. Mine have phone numbers for all over . . .'

and at times individuals would resort to more physical strategies in order to relieve tension and anxiety as in the case of this single parent of a 14-year-old who told us:

'Sometimes I can't cope. I start trembling. I tend to smash things up (. . .). I'll pick up a plate and smash it. This is what I do and I'm not going to do harm to my daughter . . .'

A rather different form of coping is bound up with invariably painful attempts on the part of the parent (usually the mother) to resolve traumatic events in their own life. Our observations parallel the findings of the MIND Stress on Women Campaign in its conclusion that there is a paucity of support and therapy services for parents who wish to tackle underlying stress from their own childhoods, and who also may suffer from not being believed on account of suffering from mental illness (MIND, 1992).

This is illustrated by the example of one mother who found herself unable to look after her 2-week-old son in the face of her mental health problem, and as a result left him in the care of her parents-in-law. Her strategy in dealing with her own distress and her son's need for explanation is revealed in this extract:

'When he got to 11 years old I knew he more or less would understand, which thank God he did. (Later) I felt relieved and happy. At the time I was telling him, I was upset and distressed, because there were personal things which I had to tell him which I didn't really want to, but I had to do to explain why he was up at (his grandparents) . . .'

However there were clearly circumstances when none of the above were any longer effective. It was when a crisis arose in a parent's mental health which could not easily be resolved; when routine or informal strategies broke down or were no longer sufficient to meet the needs of the respondent or his/her children, that professional help was sought, or brought in.

Professional responses

We should again emphasize that whilst many of our respondents mentioned a number of professionals with whom they were in contact, we were particularly interested to hear what they had to say about social workers they had encountered since they, more than other workers, were likely to have statutory responsibilities both to the parent and the child. The comments are grouped under three headings: the extent to which professionals concentrated on individual pathology as evidence of not coping; whether social workers undermined or supported parenting strengths; and the extent to which help and intervention focused on the child rather than on the parent–child relationship. While there were some positive comments, the majority of our interviewees tended to see social worker responses as intrusive and unwelcome.

Pathology focus

A major concern for these parents was the extent to which all professionals focused on the symptoms and effects of mental health problems in their work. This was seen to be excluding or marginalizing other issues such as housing and welfare benefits. The view sometimes conveyed was that symptoms and their effect on family relationships constituted the proper objects of their attention rather than material needs, which were regarded at times as not entirely acceptable demands. One father told us:

'They said we were using help from their service to try to get a house . . .'

This was not a universal view. Some respondents told us not only of getting solid practical help, but also valuing the worker's attention to the user's wish to concentrate on their mental health problem: this is what we came to call a positive/explicit pathology focus. An example of this is where the user feels they can talk openly to the social worker without being judged:

> 'I can tell my social worker things I would never think of talking to my husband about (. . .) whereas family think "oh well, never mind, just brush it off" (. . .) with the social worker you can sit down and talk and he understands how you are actually feeling.'

However, the largest grouping of responses suggested a focus on pathology which was both explicit and experienced as negative, first because it may have been felt to undermine a parent's own attempts to emphasize their caring abilities over and above their own needs. It also related to implications about the quality (or lack) of care provided and the possible risks with which the child may be faced. Both these responses could also be anticipated in a sample group of parents who are not defined as having mental health problems, but whose children are perceived to be at risk (Thorpe, 1994). We are here reminded that social workers exercise a good deal of power in the lives of those they deal with, and that service users will, with good reason, balance their emotional needs for help with their expectation of the consequences. One father (from the partnership where both parents were suffering from mental health problems) told us:

> 'I've seen how powerful they can be with (his partner). They can literally ruin your life (. . .) Telling you when you can sleep at this particular address, and when you can't. So I never tell my social worker when I've had an off-day, or when we've been up against the wall.'

Here it appears that concern about possible risk to children arising from these parents' mental health problems became the pivot of intervention and underlined the extent of their problems. We will now look at this in more detail.

Focus on strengths and weaknesses

In only three interviews were we given an unambiguous picture of professionals affirming the strengths of parents. For many of the interviewees, the actions of social workers (if not their actual words) were said to show a lack of trust in, or recognition of, parenting strengths. One mother, who said that she felt 'looked down on', sums up the tone of one-third of the interviews when she described how social workers had ignored her attempts to take what she had seen as positive steps to maintain contact with her daughter. They had concentrated, she thought, on the negative aspects of her circumstances in dissuading her from keeping her links. According to these respondents there appears to be an assumption on the part of these workers that a mental health service user who has children is *a priori* likely to have problems in satisfactory parenting. One woman remarked that:

> '(social workers) seem to think that if you've a mental health need, then your children are in danger . . .'

Focus on children

The main point to be made by almost all the users with whom we spoke is that help can come thick and fast when children are involved, but otherwise is very patchy. The point was made graphically by the father in the relationship where both partners had a mental illness:

> 'I've had a mental illness now for 8 years and in that time I never saw a social worker or a community nurse visit (. . .). As soon as our daughter was born, they were round like bees round the honeypot . . .'

Clearly when a parent is suffering mental health problems, to have your difficulties recognized only in terms of your child's safety and security is to experience a denial of your own needs. In addition there are bound to be feelings of hostility to the social worker involved. It might be argued that this emphasis arises from the child-centred statutory responsibilities which social workers exercise. We would here point out that many of our respondents were referring to a period (up to around the mid-1980s) when social work practice was still largely generic, and mental health and child care specialisms remained broadly speaking undeveloped. Indeed the Children Act 1989 was only operationalized during the period of our research (1991). Whether matters are dealt with differently as specialist teams have become established in most (though by no means all) authorities must await further research.

Giving information

We have referred earlier to the often readily available help which would come at times of crisis (or indeed over longer periods when a family member was suffering from a severe mental illness) from families, namely grandparents and siblings as well as spouses. While this would take the form of alternative care of children, particularly at times of hospital admission, a regular comment made by our informants was that their relatives (and themselves) were given inadequate explanations of the mental health problem, its likely prognosis and the effects of medication given to treat it. One woman thought that too much was assumed about her husband's ability to cope with her and their small child when she was discharged from hospital. She thought that:

> '(. . .) there should have been someone to explain things to him . . .'

The most appropriate person to take on this role may vary according to the individual task required (e.g. the psychiatrist or community psychiatric nurse might most profitably take on the task regarding illness and medication). However the most appropriate person has often been seen as the social worker (Hudson, 1982), and judging from the comments from a number of our respondents, this becomes more sharply focused as a potential task for social workers where there are children and young people involved, who may themselves be undertaking a significant amount of care of the ill parent without any (or sufficient) information about mental illness. This may well argue for an earlier and more preventative role for social workers, and other mental health professionals (Allen and Morris, 1992).

Suitability of service provision

A common thread runs through the comments made by our respondents on the access to and suitability of the range of services and facilities, that is, that services should take account of the practical realities of childcare. The timing and location of appointments, the availability of creche facilities, and the child-centredness of services in general all affected how our respondents used the services they were offered. The example we were given is that struggling on two buses each way in order to sit for what may be a long time with a toddler in a waiting room that does not contain anything to occupy the child will merely add to mental distress, and undermine any benefits of the service on offer. Realigning services to attend to these criticisms (or doing more home visits) would be relatively simple to organize, though not without a cost. A comparable point about the unsuitability of psychiatric hospital wards for family visiting was made by four of our respondents. Two of the mothers we saw told us about the extraordinary difficulties in having to care for a baby at the same time as experiencing an acute mental health crisis. This brought up the often vexed question of 'mother and baby units' and social services residential care. As one mother told us:

> 'Some people would like their babies to be in with them, wouldn't they? . . . but not in a place like this. If I was in (named ward and hospital), I wouldn't want my child to be in with me.'

Whilst the existence of dedicated units in hospitals was welcomed by some of our other respondents, the replies took us into the contentious area of parents rightly demanding more help and resources at home in order to prevent the need for hospital admission where there are small children involved.

Conclusions

Whilst it is difficult to derive neat research conclusions from the material provided by such a small-scale study, we nevertheless feel that certain key themes emerge from what our respondents told us. Primarily what these parents experienced was a recognition of their multiple and sometimes conflicting roles as parents, as service users and paradoxically as people from whom their children (according to the views of professionals) may from time to time need to be protected. Amongst the losses we saw was the diminution of meaningful time spent with or looking after the child, reduced energy levels for childcare, and in many cases a series of separations of parent and child all resulting from parental mental illness. There was to some extent a taking-on of new roles associated with supportive relationships within the family, and at times new roles such as step-parenting a new partner's children or becoming a grandparent, coinciding with periods of calm or remission in illness. We heard how one-to-one relationships with a child could become changed so that it is the child who in a reversal of roles tends to look after the needs of the parent in ways which, whilst being age-inappropriate for the child, seem to convey at times both love and a puzzled understanding of the parent's manifest distress.

The second central theme which emerged from the interviews was the criticism of professionals, who were widely seen as preoccupied with illness pathology, tending to emphasize weaknesses rather than the strengths of service users, and were perceived as focusing on the needs and protection of children to the exclusion of the linked but separate needs of the parent. To this extent social workers and other mental health professionals were seen as failing our respondents, in not giving the kind of help and support that the parents felt they most needed (advice on issues like housing and welfare benefits, or information on mental health issues, either for themselves or presented in an appropriate manner for their children).

In failing to recognize our respondents' multiple roles as parents, service users and informants about matters of mental illness, there is clearly an issue for social workers in particular in holding together these different aspects of their clients' lives, given the potentially conflicting emphases within the policy and legislation governing the role of social services departments. What social workers should guard against are the extremes in which the expressed needs of service users are forgotten, or else are assumed in themselves to be indicative of risk to their children.

A third thematic strand which came across powerfully was the inaccessibility and sometimes unsuitability of the services on offer to these parents. This included a lack of provision for children in waiting areas, lack of creche facilities and the difficulties in attending day centres and day hospitals when you are a single parent of a young child.

Postscript

In describing how he felt about the professional services his family had received, one of our respondents referred to what he called 'a lot of degrading in the name of mental health'. However we may choose to interpret that comment, there is no doubt that in the 5 years since this research was undertaken, an often polarized public debate has arisen regarding people with serious mental disorders who are living in the community (the Clunis Report: Ritchie *et al.*, 1994), with demands for additional controls over their lives in the form of supervision registers and supervised hospital discharge orders (Department of Health, Mental Patients in the Community Act, 1995).

While none of this debate has explicitly been about people who are parents, the implication is that increasingly the public has come to see the mental health patient as someone with a potential for being dangerous. In such a climate of concern, fed all too readily by media stereotypes about mental illness, it would be easy for a service user looking after his or her children to be regarded as too risky a proposition. When crises occur for them (as they inevitably will, given what our research has shown), there is a risk that they may forfeit their right to be regarded as a safe parent. Such individuals are liable to be caught in the spotlight of media prejudice and mental health professionals' uncertainty and are therefore more likely to face an interrogation of their parenting skills and family functioning, rather than the support and assistance they really need.

Acknowledgements

We would like to record our appreciation of the service users who shared their experiences so freely with us; also of the service users and professionals who assisted us in making the practical arrangements for the research. The project was funded by the Nuffield Foundation, to whom we would like to convey our thanks.

The size of the task facing professional agencies

Jennifer Bernard and Anthony Douglas

Child protection and mental health are the two highest profile social services in Britain. At least 30 enquiries are currently (April 1997) under way nationally into homicides, rapes or suicides involving people with mental health problems. When Christopher Clunis killed Jonathan Zito (Ritchie *et al.*, 1994), his action fuelled a popular view that care in the community has failed as a national policy. This echoed the child protection enquiries of the 1980s, such as into events and services in Cleveland and the Orkneys, when commentators questioned the professional calibre of British social services.

Two dismal outcomes reflect the public mood. Firstly, a lack of confidence in social work and social workers, where simultaneously and without apparent contradiction inactivity and indifference will be criticized, as will alleged interference and lack of respect for privacy and family rights. Secondly, the demonization of people with exceptionally high support needs, like Christopher Clunis, or parents defined solely as abusers.

The issues are always in the news. In 1995, a British woman, Caroline Beale, was initially charged with murder when her baby died in her care in New York. In March 1996, after 8 months in gaol, she returned to psychiatric care in Britain, having pleaded guilty to a reduced manslaughter charge. Press coverage almost incidentally revealed more and more of her distress, and the fact that she had mental health problems before and after the birth of her child.

The Woodley Inquiry (1995) was established to review the circumstances leading to the murder of a service user at an East End mental health day centre by Steven Laudat, who suffered from severe mental illness. Mr Laudat's mother had a severe mental illness, and the extent to which this pervaded family life and impacted on Steven was not fully realized by local professionals: 'My mother was mentally ill, and I was starved by her, sort of thing, and I didn't have enough to eat most of the time. I was subjected to some beatings as well from her, and nothing was done for me.' Professionals defined the situation as one where an adult with mental health problems had refused help, not as a child in need requiring help in his own right. He could have been identified as a young carer; as a child who might himself be developing mental health problems linked to inter-generational mental ill-health; and as a child suffering abuse. These factors accumulated into long-term emotional damage, although separately they may have appeared less significant.

In Ken Loach's film *Ladybird Ladybird* (Channel 4 1994), a woman 'loses' her first six children to 'Social Services'. Social workers are portrayed as victimizing her and removing child after child, even when she is living with a caring partner and her children appear safe. The actions of the social worker are depicted as persecutory, driving her and her new partner to violence and to the brink of mental illness. Research suggests that most parents fear that their children will be removed as soon as child protection concerns emerge, even when the risk is low level and there is very little chance that this will in reality happen (Department of Health, 1995a,b; Thorburn *et al.*, 1995).

Parents with a defined mental health problem will have other concerns.

'The social worker is trying to control my advice to my children. It's up to me to tell them about religion, it's not for her to try and stop me. She is too bossy. I feel like I have to shut off from them when she's around, I don't feel at ease, she don't know nothing about them except their reports. I don't like being intimidated.'

These are the words of one mother coping with manic depression making a formal complaint to a local authority.

The tensions

These examples demonstrate the tensions inherent in the work, and help to explain the complexities of achieving an appropriate level of integration between mental health and childcare services. Highly publicized failures in care have led to demands for raised standards within each service. Child protection staff and mental health staff are most likely to work in separate worlds, supported by parallel but uncoordinated guidance. Within their specialist worlds, staff can fail to see the full picture when families have multiple needs. This chapter considers how services might be brought closer together, recognizing the pressures within specialist services and the boundaries to be negotiated.

Childcare workers need mental health skills, and vice versa. There are varied and numerous interconnections that must be explored in working with a child or adult, separately or as part of a family group. The mental health problems of a parent will require consideration of the needs of the family for support and of the children for care and protection. In a few cases, the standard of assessment and care planning work will be scrutinized by a Family Proceedings Court or a guardian *ad litem*. The mental health problems of a child will require consideration of the origins of his or her distress, and the needs of the family for support because of the impact of the child's behaviour. Adult or child carers warrant special concern, and their needs are likely to require an assessment under the Carers (Recognition and Services Act), which became law on 1 April 1996. Adult survivors of abuse may have mental health problems, and child victims of abuse may develop mental health problems. Either may go on to abuse others.

Research demonstrates the increased risk of child psychiatric disorder when parents have mental health problems, notably maternal depression (Brown and Harris, 1978; AMA, 1993). In one study, over half of the children with mild to severe behavioural problems had mothers who were significantly depressed, whilst this was the case in only 3.3 per cent of children without problems. The rate of depression in a group of mothers of school children in an outer London Borough in 1977 was found to be about 30 per cent.

An American study of families seen at a parenting clinic intended to improve the ability of families to cope with very difficult child behaviour, identified the possible links between parental stress and abuse (Whipple and Webster-Stratton, 1991). It concluded that parental stress was an important factor in precipitating abuse, with mothers under stress relating this to life events and displaying higher rates of depression and anxiety. Families where physical abuse was used were significantly more often in receipt of low incomes, had younger mothers with less education, more often reported family histories involving abuse, and were more likely to be abusing alcohol or drugs. Children from abusive households had significantly more behavioural problems. It may be that families with these characteristics were more likely to use the service offered by the parenting clinic, or be referred to it, although the study did include families described as middle class and with healthy incomes. Over 90 per cent of the parents were Caucasian.

In British terms, the children of parents with severe mental health problems, intermittent or enduring, are very likely to be children in need within the scope of the Children Act. One study showed that half of the children of parents with formally diagnosed psychotic illness had evidence of emotional and behavioural problems (Falkov, 1996 quoted in Rickford, 1996a). This does not mean that all parents with mental health problems are poor parents, or that children cannot cope with parents who are unstable or unpredictable. The evidence is, however that children in these circumstances are either over-aware of their parents moods, or will have to care for or withdraw from their parents more than an average child would. The adverse affects are well catalogued (Richman, 1977; Sheppard, 1993). The definition of these children as 'in need' should ensure that their care and development is kept under review independently of the requirements of their parents.

Webster (1990) reports that particular care will be required in assessing the needs of the children of women with a diagnosis of schizophrenia. As women tend to develop the condition later, they are more likely to be parents than men with the condition. She explores the consequences of separation for these children from their parents, and concludes that support for fathers (and the extended family of fathers) is important to the well-being of the children. It is now known that the children of parents with schizophrenia have a genetic predisposition to the condition which may be triggered by life events. The difficulties associated with separate placements are enhanced for these children, particularly when contact with parents is emotionally charged and not mediated by the normality of domestic tasks. It is nonetheless important to ensure that any delusional state of either parent is not harmful to the child, in terms of their physical as well as their emotional safety. The implications for local authorities are that staff, including residential childcare staff or foster carers, who may be involved in the episodic or longer term care of children in such circumstances, are alert to the care required to minimize the likelihood of the child's future mental health being compromised. Family aide support or the consistent use of the same foster carer will be the most helpful, if assistance from outside the family is required.

Murder is still rare in Britain. The victims are most likely to be members of the murderer's family, and this holds true for homicides where the murderer had a severe mental illness. Of the 12 English women in the sample considered by the Confidential Inquiry Into Homicides and Suicides by Mentally Ill People, nine had killed their own children aged between 10 days and 13 years. Eight of these nine women had been diagnosed as suffering from a depressive illness, one from a personality disorder. All 12 were outpatients at the time of the murder. Of the 27 English men in the sample who had murdered, 14 of the victims had been from their own family, although the age of the victims is not specified.

The incidence of serious mental illness in children is also rare, but an estimated 10 to 20 per cent of children will 'at some time have a mental health problem which will require help' (Department of Health, 1995c). Factors cited as affecting the likelihood of developing mental health problems include family disadvantage; family discord or separation; a parent with a mental illness; poor parenting; chronic physical illness in the child; some chromosomal or genetic abnormalities; brain damage in the child; physical, sexual or emotional abuse; sudden or extreme trauma; and learning disability or language or communication problems.

There is American evidence that of young people diagnosed as requiring inpatient or substantial outpatient tertiary psychiatric care, a high proportion (41 per cent) had some form of inappropriate sexual behaviours, including victimization (Adams *et al.*, 1995). Of this group, 82 per cent had a history of having been sexually abused. Having been abused was not a necessary or sufficient predictor of abusive behaviour, however. There was a predictive link between the chronicity of the abuse and the number of abusers, those most severely abused being those most likely to offend against others. The authors suggest that this highlights the need for early detection and intervention with abused children to seek to prevent future abusive behaviour. Such intervention would include appropriate techniques with adult perpetrators of abuse, and therefore close links with the criminal justice agencies, and particularly the Probation Service where work has been done on the characteristics and techniques of adult offenders (Northumbria Probation Service Sex Offenders Team and the Department of Adolescent Forensic Psychiatry, Newcastle Mental Health Trust 1994). It is suggested that British work lags far behind that done in America and the Netherlands (King, 1988). Providing a therapeutic service to young abusers also falls within this category.

A failure to intervene effectively with children will affect the mental health of the next generation of adults. If child and adolescent mental health services 'are inadequate in their planning or in their delivery, they permit continued suffering among young people and their families and allow a continuing spiral of child abuse, juvenile crime, family breakdown and adult mental health problems' (Health Advisory Service, 1995).

In other areas of specialist work, considerations of the mental health dimension of a service user's needs is important. For instance, women who have placed their children for adoption may develop mental health problems many years after the event, with feelings of guilt, loss and low self-esteem. Hughes and Logan (1995) conclude that 'Parting with a child had a profound impact on the mental health of some birth mothers.'

The guidance

Until very recently, reviews of mental health services or guidance for mental health staff made not a single mention of childcare concerns and how they might be handled. The publication of *Building Bridges* in 1996 (Department of Health, 1996a) has finally put into print the recognition that teams will need to 'build up links' with child protection services. Even this reference focuses on child protection and risk assessment, rather than child development or the possibility of children in need being part of a family where the adult is ill. The 38 competencies by which social workers are assessed for approval under the 1983 Mental Health Act contain no mention of skills in family work or awareness of child protection issues. Similarly, child protection guidance makes no mention of the skills needed to work with a parent with mental health difficulties.

Specialisms

If communication between staff or agencies is poor, or the knowledge base of professionals is weak, risks to both children and their parents inevitably increase.

Child protection work and mental health work may both involve cases which require a speedy professional response. In agencies without adequate working arrangements between specialist services, the mental health staff member may be unable to obtain a quick response from the local childcare team because the mental health emergency may not appear to be a child protection one. Similarly, a childcare team may try to arrange for an approved social work assessment of a family member, believing that parental mental health problems are critical to family functioning. To the mental health team, those problems may seem minor and not constitute an emergency. At its worst, action can take days or even weeks to negotiate between the relevant teams.

It may then be left to the out-of-hours services to resolve the issues, prompted by the anxieties of one group of staff or the direct action of another agency experiencing delays in following up referrals made through conventional routes. Interestingly, out-of-hours duty social workers and directors of social services may soon be the only generic staff left in local social services departments, as day-time services all become specialist.

Having said this, we would consider it a retrograde step to return to the era before specialization, when for many authorities mental health services received a very low priority relative to the all-encompassing and voracious demands of the childcare services. Since April 1993 when the community care changes were introduced, services that were previously barely visible, such as those for substance misusers or people with HIV/AIDS, have gained more status and perhaps a fairer share of resources. Certainly there is likely to be more professional and even public interest because of their inclusion in community care plans. The generic approach may have concealed unacceptable variations in levels of services and standards of practice as well as distorted priorities.

If vulnerable children or adults do fall through the gaps between specialist services which are operating in parallel rather than jointly, the consequences may be literally fatal. Falkov (1996) suggests that between one-quarter and three-quarters of fatal child abuse within the family is perpetrated by a parent with a psychiatric disorder. Parental mental illness was detected in a third of the 100 Part 8 Review reports for the two years (1993 and 1994) that he studied, where children had died. As Hunter Johnston's (1996) covering letter to Falkov's study states, 'The study concludes that professionals working with children need to develop greater awareness of the effect of parental mental health on children and that in adult services a child welfare and protection perspective needs to be incorporated into assessment and treatment.'

Two case studies known to the authors, neither the subject of a Part 8 Review, illustrate this theme. In the first, a man known locally as a model father killed his child in the middle of the night. Just before the murder, he began to chant and became highly agitated. Afterwards, there was some concern that the anabolic steroids he had been taking as part of a fanatical fitness regime may have induced a temporary psychosis. Four years earlier, there was an entry in his GP's records expressing concern about his mental health and possible paranoid tendencies. There was no inter-agency communication about this man and his family.

In the second family, a young man aged 17 years is most likely to have killed a baby being looked after by his mother, an unregistered child-minder. He is thought to have set the house alight to disguise the murder. The young man and his mother escaped the fire. There was insufficient evidence to charge him. Throughout his 20s he lived with a series of women, all of whom he assaulted repeatedly. Most of them did not report this domestic violence. This information remained on separate files in the records of the police, the Domestic Violence Unit and health visitors. He also attended a number of psychiatric emergency clinics around London, but was never formally assessed. One night, aged 27 years, in a rage, he took his 5-year-old daughter down to the Thames and threw her in the river. It is almost certain that the man had displayed unrecognized symptoms of mental disorder since his own childhood. Could the murder of the two children in these cases have been averted?

The combination of a parent with severe mental health problems and a child who may be in need of protection demands an almost impossibly high level of skill in risk assessment and decision making. The mainstream government response has been to establish lists of potentially abusive adults – child protection registers for children most at risk, in the main from their families, and supervision registers for adults with mental health problems who pose grave risks to the public (or themselves).

Registers do not in themselves offer protection. They are not linked. They are maintained by different agencies. There are different decision-making processes required for names to be added to them. Their main weakness is that whilst they should reflect an accurate historical record of past violence or risk, they cannot be used to predict future dangers with any degree of certainty. The main strength of registers is that they should at a minimum ensure that there is explicit responsibility for keeping in touch with individuals or families, and, most importantly, ensuring that if they move around, information moves with them to their new statutory agencies.

Assessment

Literature can advise assessors that an adult who abuses a child is in general terms more likely to be depressed; to have been abused; to have run away from home or had a disrupted family life; to have got into fights as a child; to be more emotionally dependent, more drug dependent and more alcohol dependent; to be more tense, more hostile and less mature than a non-abusing adult. (Brown and Harris, 1976; Taylor *et al.*, 1991; Adams *et al.*,1995). These general findings cannot help social workers predict which adults in which circumstances will become abusive. Indeed the adult may not have been identified as a 'client' on the basis of these factors by any single agency.

The links between mental health problems and the predictors of child abuse are even weaker. Depression, personality disorders, poor learning skills, and emotional disorders have been identified in various studies (Brown and Harris, 1976; Taylor *et al.*, 1991; Falkov, 1995). Health and social care staff are like detectives, searching for a sustainable hypothesis, looking for hard facts in each unique case. Again, these characteristics would not necessarily by themselves lead to the recognition by any agency of a significant potential problem in childcare.

There is a danger that professional anxieties become heightened by behaviour defined as anti-social, such as drug misuse, or asking for help because of mental health problems. The risks to children may become overstated. Professional systems may undermine parents struggling to cope with their own mental health problems and minimize the disruptive consequences, or add to stress by investigation rather than providing family support. A parent believed to have neglected or abused a child may be set very high targets for behavioural change, to convince the professionals involved that future harm will be avoided. Unrealistic targets for change can be daunting and bewildering, and may cause parents to give up their hopes of carrying on caring, prematurely. The weight of professional anxiety or the impact of negative labelling may cause childcare staff with a limited understanding of mental illness to act precipitously in removing children from the care of their parents.

Other factors may increase the labelling effect. MIND's Policy Paper (1993) on women and mental health summarizes the 'enormous obstacles' women face in becoming mentally healthy adults, the difficulties in having the causes of their distress recognized, and the costs of entry into the mental health system. Among MIND's recommendations are the recognition of the caring responsibilities of many women, and better childcare services for women needing day, residential or in-patient care – including services where small children can also be accommodated (MIND, 1993). Difficulties with appropriate treatment where women may have children also arise for misusers of drugs and alcohol. It is suggested by voluntary agencies that rehabilitation services are designed for men without childcare responsibilities and that women residents are likely to be in the minority which can lead to additional harassment or even abuse (Release, 1995). The same criticism has been made by MIND of psychiatric facilities. Fear of children being removed is cited as being a major factor deterring women from seeking treatment. This emphasizes another common link between child protection services and mental health services, in that many women fear the consequences of seeking help from either.

Parents from black or minority ethnic communities, particularly if they are poor or a lone parent, may face additional discrimination. Black mothers may be in quadruple jeopardy, facing discrimination for being black, being a woman, having a mental health problem and being perceived as inherently more likely to chastize or neglect a child. Black men are overrepresented in the population detained in psychiatric care. If the first language of a parent is not English, there will be additional complications, even with the assistance of skilled interpreters who understand mental health issues, and mental health and childcare law and practice.

One local authority, Kent Social Services, developed a special training programme for community interpreters who needed these particular skills.

Sexual orientation may also be a factor leading to discriminatory behaviour. Gay men with mental health problems may not get sympathetic or knowledgeable care or treatment, and the possibility of them having been abused is often overlooked. Lesbian mothers, or bisexual fathers, may be perceived as unsatisfactory parents. Gay men are often misunderstood as being more likely to be paedophiles than heterosexual men.

Agencies seeking to recognize and minimize the effects of discrimination, and to avoid discriminatory behaviour by their staff, must ensure their staff are trained and secure in anti-discriminatory practice. This may be politically and publicly contentious. Staff themselves may find it difficult to consider issues of sexuality, gender or race and will need to feel secure in the support of their agencies. White men still form a significant majority in senior management in all agencies, and in most professions, particularly the medical profession. It may be more difficult for them to provide the necessary reassurances, or to be sensitive to the staff and service issues involved.

It is also important to recognize the strengths of families who have coped successfully with long-term mental health problems, and not just their difficulties. Sometimes these strengths can be put to good effect for others. At least one adoption panel to our knowledge has approved a couple to adopt where the male partner suffered from schizophrenia. Following a lengthy assessment, which included medical recommendations, it was decided that the strengths of the couple, including their experience of coping successfully with schizophrenia, meant that they would be very suitable adopters for a particular child.

The strengths and benefits of involving 'survivors' of mental health problems in service delivery as well as service planning are well recognized. The involvement of parents who have been subjects of childcare or child protection referrals is standard practice for some authorities when they plan services and train staff.

Joint working

It is not the intention of this chapter to dwell on the well-understood difficulties in working together between professions and across agencies. What is of concern is the fragmentation of purchasing arrangements for services as a consequence of cross-boundary contracting by health authorities for specialist services and the advent of GP fund-holding and commissioning. Where fund-holding or commissioning is in place, social workers have had to secure agreements from GPs to make referrals to core services such as child and family consultation (formerly child guidance clinics). A GP may fund care for the parent with a mental health problem, but require the local authority to meet the costs of care for the accompanying child. The macro-purchasing responsibilities of health authorities are now devolved to micro-purchasers. Within slimmed down health authorities, expertise is scarce on specialist areas of health contracting. The situation with primary care groups may well be the same.

A recent report has identified the extent to which inpatient psychiatric care is now provided within the independent sector, particularly for behavioural work. The Sainsbury Centre for Mental Health analysed the data for 1994 and identified that one in six of acute psychiatric facilities are provided for within the independent sector, with a possible 23 per cent of the independent sector places available being paid for by the NHS. The NHS payments were almost entirely funded by health authorities as extra-contractual referrals (Warner and Ford, 1996). This phenomenon raises some difficult questions as few, if any, local authorities provide a social work service to the independent sector. Depending on the location of the unit, care planning, particularly for discharge, may be extremely difficult. Of particular relevance will be how familiar the independent providers are with childcare and child protection issues, and how and to whom they would provide any information revealed during treatment or family visits. These issues should be addressed by local authorities with the health authorities as part of the contractual protocols in use with such providers.

Within local authorities, changed management arrangements for schools have also resulted in fragmentation. Child protection matters are the responsibility of local schools, and the exclusion of pupils from school is increasing. Violent or seriously disruptive behaviour in the classroom cannot be ignored, but the consequences of exclusion for children and their families are severe. Exclusion is linked with family breakdown and the possibility of social services care. Excluded children have very little formal education, and lack the maturing influences of social interaction within a formal organization. They are also more likely to be involved in youth crime (Audit Commission, 1996). Preventing exclusion from school wherever possible is to be preferred, given the fragmented educational services excluded children often receive subsequently.

Since April 1997, all local agencies have been required to cooperate in the production of a Children's Services Plan. There is a specific requirement to include details of services for children and young people with mental health problems, which reflects the Priorities and Planning Guidance for the NHS on comprehensive services for severely mentally ill people. Child protection is located within a model of family support for children, and there is a requirement that the ACPC Annual Report should form part of the Children's Services Plan. The statutory nature of the Plan should enable authorities to ensure that all prospective partners in care participate. The introduction of statutory community care plans, where services for adults with a mental health problem are identified, has at least helped to make transparent the resources available to meet identified need, and unarguable gaps in services. Whilst it would not be possible for one document to serve every purpose, child protection and mental health concerns will be found in the Children's Services Plan, Community Care Plan, Community Care Charter and the intended Mental Health Services Charter, to name only those of immediate relevance. It is to be hoped that agendas rise to the challenge of ensuring that they are not only compatible but adequately cross referenced.

At an individual level, agencies have to reconcile three separate care planning processes – those required for child protection (and possibly again for childcare), care management and the care programme approach. *Building Bridges* (Department of Health, 1996a) tackles the integration of care management and the care programme approach, but there is no formal guidance on managing an integrated assessment of joint risks to family members. Within local authorities, there may be scope for further difficulties if specialist children's services do not follow a care management approach and mental health specialist services do. The impact will depend on how the authority has interpreted care management. In practice, whilst the procedural constraints may prove time-consuming, provided that a clear focus is maintained on the purpose of each care plan, within whatever system, and the way in which it links with the care plans of other members of the family, this can be overcome.

A helpful approach may be to map referral routes to existing services for family support, childcare, child protection, child and adolescent psychiatric services, youth justice and adult mental health services. This will obviously clarify the staff involved and the mechanisms used to gatekeep referrals and then respond effectively. It should also allow there to be some consideration of whether referrals are always following the most appropriate routes. What, for example, are the differences between young people in the youth justice system, psychiatric system, child and family consultation or care system? Would the outcomes for them be better if these characteristics were more specifically considered when making or accepting referrals?

The difficulty of establishing effective joint arrangements cannot be underestimated. If it was easy everyone would be doing it. When put into practice, the results may be disappointing. A study of the implementation of the Care Programme Approach in West Lambeth showed little evidence of improved outcomes for patients with marked social turbulence and a history of violence. Three-year programme results showed no significant improvement in social skills or clinical functioning. Of the patients in the original cohort, 60 per cent had subsequently been charged with violent offences, and half of the patients in the study had been victims of various crimes. There had been a massive increase in demand for services, particularly the use of hospital beds, resulting in budgetary overspends.

The final constraint on the development of practice and joint working to be considered is resources. Few local authorities or health authorities have escaped either a drip-drip or big-bang reduction in their budgets between the late 1980s and 1997. These pressures look set to continue for the rest of the decade irrespective of any change in central government. Formally, local authorities and health authorities are required to demonstrate how they target those potential service users in greatest need, particularly in mental health. In childcare and child protection, there is an emphasis on identifying serious risk but it is now balanced by a requirement to identify resources for children in need and to consider the impact of a child protection investigation in the context of family support rather than action against abusers. The benefits of social support, particularly in a crisis, are often underestimated. They include information and advice, practical help and emotional support. The approach relies more upon the provision of building blocks for good parenting, which may be missing.

Despite the de-regulation drive of successive Conservative Governments up to 1997, during the same period there was a proliferation of monitoring exercises and formal inspections of services locally and nationally through the Social Services Inspectorate, National Health Service Executive, Health Advisory Service, Mental Health Act Commission and the Audit Commission. A feature of the separate strands of regulatory activity in central government was unfortunately that many of these exercises were carried out only in one agency by one specialist inspection team. Good inter-agency practice remains hard to identify or replicate.

Organizational arrangements

The first step towards better outcomes for adults and children is to identify the potential problems. These can be summarized as failure to recognize the links between mental health and child protection because of specialization; poor professional practice in risk assessment and care planning; and limited inter-agency commissioning and service delivery mechanisms.

The Health Advisory Service developed a useful model for a strategic approach to commissioning and delivering a comprehensive child and adolescent mental health service (Health Advisory Service, 1995). This is reproduced as Appendix 11.1. It could be adapted as a model for other specialisms, but it lacks cross reference to adult mental health or child protection, because of the focus of the original publication.

A common or shared diagnostic framework between child and adult psychiatrists might increase the detection of serious mental health problems in children and young people. This is especially important where a childhood disturbance is linked to bullying of younger children, sexualized behaviour, or self-injury, and where these child or adolescent behaviours are likely to intensify on becoming a parent or living with a child. At present both child and adolescent psychiatrists are understandably more concerned about challenging behaviour in the present than underlying factors. It cannot be right, however, that these trends are only of historic interest when a life is being pieced together at an official inquiry after a serious incident has taken place.

Local authorities should develop clear protocols for communication between specialist childcare teams and specialist mental health teams, based upon a system of named lead assessors for allocated cases, and named officers who have a liaison responsibility for unallocated cases. Such protocols ensure that cases are always discussed between specialist teams, and that clear decisions are reached at crucial stages. Without formal procedures, it is unlikely that communication between specialist teams will reach the required level of clarity. An example of such a protocol, from the London Borough of Hackney, is reproduced below. The procedure is shown as Appendix 11.2, the flow chart as Appendix 11.3. Similar protocols from Richmond ACPC (Appendix 11.4) and Kingston ACPC (Appendix 11.5) are also appended as good practice examples.

Hackney's procedure recognizes that each specialist team will routinely need to draw upon the expertise of the other, and that formal channels of communication are essential. Liaison is set at senior practitioner level, with provision for more senior managers to arbitrate if necessary. An emphasis is placed on joint approaches, particularly joint assessment. The procedure stipulates that no allocated family case held by either team can be closed without joint managerial say-so and the consent of the responsible psychiatrist. Common geographical boundaries help such arrangements, whereby at least the community health trust and local authority work to the same boundaries. It is unfortunate that local government reorganization and health commissioning reorganization have not paid more attention to common boundaries for health and social care.

Protocols such as Hackney's (and Richmond and Kingston's) need backing up with joint training for childcare workers and mental health workers. Training should help staff to avoid polarized attitudes, such as crusading for the parent and avoiding the needs and rights of the child, or failing to appreciate that the well-being of the child is usually best furthered by remaining within a well-supported birth family, however perilous that can sometimes seem. Training should also ensure that in complex cases staff undertake a comprehensive and multi-professional assessment and care plan, not two separate assessments which are then left to a case conference to choose between. There will, however, be a requirement to satisfy the statutory planning processes for child protection and for mental health within this joint approach. Care must also be taken that the two sets of staff do not engage in a power struggle about their respective importance but see their roles as enabling the organization to take a more rounded approach to the needs of each family as a whole.

To be successful, training programmes need to be carried out within a clear operational policy which emphasizes at a formal level that social services departments and health trusts, in particular, are aware of the overlaps between childcare and mental health professional practice. Within this policy, the prioritization of cases should be encouraged where concerns may last for many years, not least through a review system which ensures that families are kept in touch with, monitored and offered as much support as possible within finite resources.

Training must also recognize that local authority in-house residential and day services will on occasion look after parents with mental health problems and/or their children, even when they are not designated as specialist resources. Care might be provided in family centres, or day nurseries, mental health resource centres, children's homes, with child-minders and foster carers or almost anywhere. Sometimes this reflects the lack of a specialist resource, sometimes flexibility in particular circumstances and a wish to remain in full control of the assessment and the management of a care plan. Much unheralded preventative and care work is carried out in this way, when counselling, group work, therapy and basic advice and support may be on offer to parents and children.

Authorities should give consideration to ensuring that there is at least one social worker in each childcare or child protection team who is an approved social worker, and that one social worker in each mental health team is experienced in child protection work. Similar arrangements should be considered where other specialisms overlap, such as mental health and learning disability, or childcare and substance misuse.

For over 20 years, inter-agency child protection services have been overseen by Area Child Protection Committees (ACPCs). Their capacity for action is limited by not having direct control over the agencies under their umbrella, but they have acted as a forum for inter-agency case reviews, training and practice development. At the same time, academic and professional research, especially in the 1990s, has helped to redefine child protection work within a broader childcare service. The need for structured family support, services for young carers, services for young abusers, and parenting programmes, is now widely recognized. The recognition of the imperative of strong inter-agency cooperation, which has emerged as a recommendation from virtually every child protection inquiry, has gained further momentum, if it needed it, from the requirement to produce a children's services plan. On top of this, the inquiries keep coming, only the most sensational now attracting public attention.

There has been no formal government consideration of the possible benefits of creating a local forum for inter-agency mental health working, similar to that provided through the ACPCs or Drug Action Teams (which are the responsibility of the District Health Authorities to set up). Some authorities have set up action teams for making an impact on joint development. Wirral Health and Wirral Social Services, for example, reviewed all adult mental health services in wide consultation with users, carers and service providers. Others have standing advisory groups as part of their joint planning processes, such as Newcastle-upon-Tyne. Clear local demarcation between planning groups is essential in the absence of an integrated national structure.

Service options

Sometimes children living in extremely unsatisfactory circumstances, subjected to long-term abuse and a disrupted pattern of care, should be offered an alternative family to live in. However, childcare teams should always consider long-term family support rather than an apparently more straightforward alternative. Family support plans may be costly, but so is hospital care for the parent (or child) or local authority care for the child (or parent). The experiences and outcomes for children moving into foster or adoptive care remain uncertain. This approach may not be well understood by mental health staff, although they would also be seeking to avoid compulsory admission to hospital.

An example of a complex and tense multi-agency and multidisciplinary family support package illustrates the issues. A young couple were expecting a child. They lived together, near to the woman's parents in an urban area – she had not been diagnosed as having a defined mental illness, but was under psychiatric supervision as a condition of a Probation Order. This was because of the unexplained murder of her first child at or very shortly after birth, whilst she was in the bathroom at her parent's home. The baby had been stabbed repeatedly, but neither the mother nor anyone else in the household accepted responsibility. The mother had no memory of the child's death. The couple wanted to keep their child. The psychiatric evaluation of risk was ambivalent because of the unacknowledged circumstances of the death of the first child. The paediatric evaluation favoured close assessment of the couple as parents after the birth but could offer no inpatient assessment services as staff on the most appropriate ward did not feel they could offer close enough supervision. Care proceedings would not be supported. The probation officer tended towards early removal of the child. The midwife and the health visitor were cautious. In the end, social services was left providing residential assessment in a flat attached to a mental health hostel, using a mix of mental health and childcare staff, with health visitor support. The parents were never left alone with their child during the initial assessment period, and the care plan became the subject of family court proceedings because of the anxieties of the guardian *ad litem* about the safety of the baby. Despite the considerable stresses of such close supervision, the baby thrived with its parents and was not removed. The cost of the assessment and care package was considerable.

Very few authorities are known to have established a dedicated preventative service for parents with mental health support needs and their children together. One such centre, the Wallington Resource Centre in Sutton, works with up to 15 parents and their children at any one time. The Centre is a mental health day resource centre, and has a specialist nursery for parents with children to use. The work with parents and children occupies about 20 per cent of the Centre's overall work. The St Helier NHS Trust and Sutton Social Services fund the Centre.

All parents meet the criteria for the Care Programme Approach in their own right, and the nursery supports children from 0–5 years of age. Following school admission, the Centre continues to offer long-term support for parents. Day care is seen as essential provision for these parents, and women using the Centre also make use of peer support for baby-sitting and other help during crises. Individual support is also available through therapy, family groups and other programmes. The service has been operating for over 20 years, and also offers a service to parents who have outpatient appointments or other commitments related to their illness with no childcare arrangements to cover them. Most local authorities make *ad hoc* arrangements for placements for children whose parents have mental health problems, but it is rare to provide an integrated specialist service which recognizes the long-term nature of the commitment to each family and caters for their separate needs.

Barnardos Willow Project in Leeds provides a counselling service and organizes outings and other activities for children of 5 years of age upwards who have a severely mentally ill parent. The first contact for children with the Project may come after a family crisis when a parent has a hospital admission. The Project Coordinator described a 12-year-old girl with two schizophrenic parents who, after 18 months' involvement with the Project, started to mention worries about her mother walking around all night and describing events which the child knew had not happened. 'They don't see themselves as young carers, because this is all they have known. Sometimes they take on the parent's reality and lose trust in their own judgement' (Rickford, 1996a).

Salford Community Health Trust health visitors wanted to identify mothers who were suffering from postnatal depression and might need extra support. They used a recognized assessment scale with the mothers of children up to 8 weeks old and were surprised at the high incidence of postnatal depression revealed. Within the same service, a sleep clinic is offered to parents who have children with poor sleeping patterns. This is in recognition of the impact of difficult behaviour on the mental health of all the members of the family. A specifically designed programme using behavioural techniques is put in place for each family.

Other specific projects can be targeted positively at parents with mental health support needs. The Mother and Baby Unit at the Queen's Medical Centre at Nottingham University assesses women experiencing severe postnatal depression and chronic schizophrenia. It offers a day and inpatient service on a continuous assessment basis for periods of up to 2 months. Community follow-up is organized until the mother is well again or until the baby is 1 year old and past the most dangerous time for a child at risk of physical abuse (Thompson, 1995).

In Newham, the Area Child Protection Committee is using a jointly developed definition to monitor the number of children coming through the formal child protection case conference system where either they or their parents or carers have mental health support needs. This information will be used to inform the commissioning of services. The initiative was stimulated by the recommendations from the Woodley Inquiry. The Newham ACPC is also considering the therapeutic needs of children whose parents have mental health support needs.

Conclusion

Child protection and mental health services are arguably the most visible, vulnerable and volatile public services in Britain. The stakes are high, with severe injury or loss of liberty the possible outcomes of professional error. In this context, the absence of national standards to guide professional practice is noteworthy. In Britain, an inexperienced and even unqualified social care worker could be allocated child protection work or users with severe mental health problems. This may be unlikely in practice, but keeping experienced staff in operational posts remains difficult, with the options for promotion to management or leaving the profession for an easier and equally well-paid alternative. Even with regular and good quality supervision, staff may be asked to manage situations for which they do not have sufficient personal or professional training or experience (Zito Trust, 1995).

By way of contrast, in the United States, the National Association of Social Workers certifies social workers who have achieved a defined professional standard. Virtually all states also licence or certify professional social workers. The authors take the view that an integrated post-qualifying accreditation system for social workers should be established, within an overall regulatory regime such as the proposed General Social Care Council.

Staff should reach these standards before carrying out high level child protection or mental health social work. An understanding of child protection and adult mental health practice issues and perspectives should be a core module for each accreditation. Where lives may be at stake, the current system is simply not good enough.

Appendix 11.1 A strategic approach to commissioning and delivering a comprehensive child and adolescent mental health service

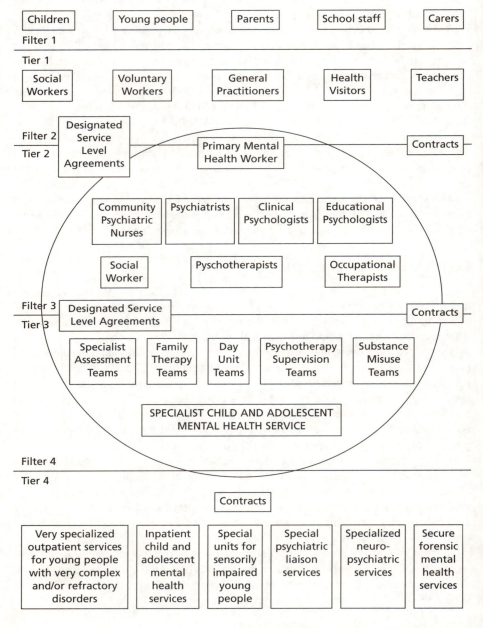

Appendix 11.2 Protocol for liaison between specialist teams in the London Borough of Hackney

1. Referral to locality mental health team of parent(s)/carer(s) with dependent children
2. Check if known to children and families division
3. Assessment by locality mental health worker
4. Consultation with supervisor
5. If concerns about care of the children in any way – consult with senior practitioner (mental health)
6. Lead practitioner (mental health) consults with the designated senior practitioner (children and families)
7. Referral to children and families division for assessment of childcare needs. This work must be prioritized
8. Referral to children and families division for urgent action, i.e. children being accommodated. This work must be prioritized
9. Planning meeting to be organized by senior practitioner (mental health) within 7 days, chaired by locality team manager or deputy
10. Planning meeting decides whether case should be allocated in children and families division. Allocation of locality worker. Planning meeting should include consultant psychiatrist
11. Case cannot be closed by children and families division unless agreed at reconvened planning meeting chaired by locality team manager or deputy, where the children and families division representative is present
12. If no concerns about child protection, case is referred to children and families division for information. Recorded by designated senior practitioner (children and families)
13. All people with a mental health problem who are carers of dependent children must have an allocated worker in the locality mental health team. These cases cannot be closed without the agreement to do so of the locality mental health team manager and the consultant psychiatrist
14. Locality mental health team manager to ensure a register system is kept which identifies those cases that require regular review

Appendix 11.3 Referral to locality team of parent/carer with dependent children – London Borough of Hackney

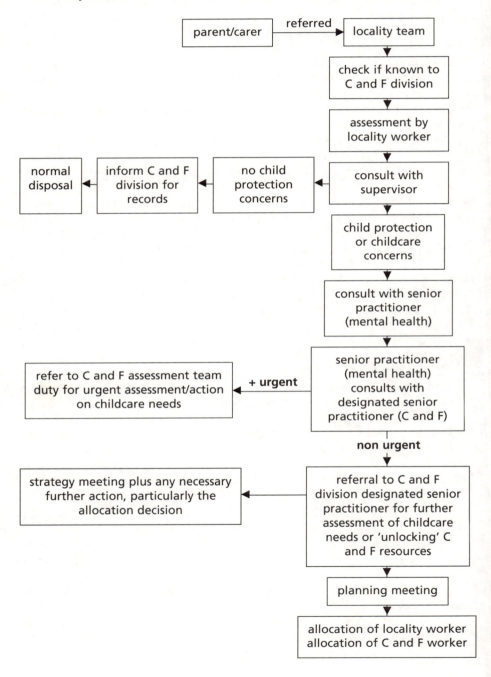

Appendix 11.4 Working in partnership

A protocol for collaborative inter-agency work in adult mental health and child protection

Published by the London Borough of Richmond Upon Thames ACPC

It is recognised that there may be occasions where there is an apparent conflict of interest between the needs of children and the needs of parents/carers with mental health problems. All agencies agree that if a child is potentially at risk of significant harm as the result of acts of commission or omission on the part of the parent/carer, **then the welfare of the child will be paramount.**

This protocol provides guidance on policy and practice with the aim of facilitating effective communication and interagency working between childrens' and adults' services, and to ensure that the welfare needs of both children and parents/carers with mental health needs are addressed.

The emphasis of these guidelines is on preventing the disruption of families and on working together to support and maintain the family unit.

This protocol should be read in conjunction with the LBRUT Area Child Protection Committee's child protection procedures and guidelines and individual agencies' policies and procedures.

1. All agencies involved in assessing whether a parent/carer has a mental illness, or in providing support to parents/carers who have been diagnosed as having a mental illness or personality disorder, should make enquiries as to whether there are children in that particular household.
2. Equally, all agencies involved in assessing the needs of children in a family should consider whether a parent/carer has mental health needs.
3. Based on the information thus collated, a decision should be reached as to whether it is necessary to undertake a more detailed assessment. Advice may be sought from a range of professionals. (See *List of Useful Contacts* [not reproduced here])
4. Consideration should be given as to whether the parent/carer's illness or disorder could adversely impact on their ability to care appropriately for any children in the household. This should take into account other support systems available, including partners, extended family members and other statutory or voluntary agencies which may be involved with the family.
5. In particular, consideration should be given to an appropriate referral if a pregnant woman or her partner has a diagnosed mental disorder.
6. **Where information suggests immediate danger to the child, there should be no delay in referring concerns (as per individual agency child protection procedures).**
7. **In extreme cases of immediate danger to life or limb, it may be necessary to notify the police. (See *List of Useful Contacts*.)**
8. Where information suggests no immediate risk to the child, consideration should then be given – in consultation with the parent/carer – to approaching other childcare agencies to arrange preventative support services.

9. Consideration should always be given to referring the family to services for children and families for support. Unless the parent/carer specifically requests that no contact be made, services for children and families will then assess what level of support can be offered.
10. Where the child is under five years of age, or is disabled, consideration should be given to contacting the family's health visitor to discuss what support is available. Where a child is of school age, consideration should be given to contacting the school nurse and/or named teacher.
11. Where there are concerns about the mental well-being of a parent/carer, advice should be sought from the appropriate community mental health team (see *List of Useful Contacts*) or via the general practitioner.
12. It is essential that throughout this process there is coordination of both services and professionals involved with the family to ensure good communication and clarity of roles. This should always include regular contact between all agencies and, where appropriate, invitations to planning/strategy meetings and Care Programme Approach reviews for all professionals involved with the family.
13. Whilst there might be some occasions where client confidentiality must be respected, every effort should be made to obtain the family's consent for information to be shared amongst agencies. Ultimately the welfare of the child will take precedence over confidentiality if there is risk of significant harm.
14. Where services for children and families are involved with a family, primary responsibility for the welfare of children in the family will remain with the locality social worker. The locality social worker will coordinate support services and should be supported in this role by all agencies working with the family.
15. Where a parent/carer is under the care of a community mental health team, responsibility for the adult only will remain with the team in question.

Useful information

ACPC Guidelines
Local agency child protection procedures
Care Programme Approach (community care for adults)
Mental Health Act Code of Practice
Children Act 1989, Guidance and Regulations
Directory of local general practitioners and health visitors.

Appendix 11.5 Mental health and children and families services: a joint protocol for assessment and care management of parental mental health problems – London Borough of Kingston-upon-Thames ACPC

1. Purpose of the protocol

- To improve coordination and communication between the family support teams and the community mental health teams in cases of parental mental illness.
- To provide for joint assessments of parents with mental health problems who are already known or are new referrals to community mental health teams or the family support teams.
- To provide integrated services to these families that are both effective and well coordinated.
- To provide a framework for planning and undertaking the joint assessment of risk for ASW Assessments under the 1983 Mental Health Act and Child Protection Assessments under the Children Act 1989.

2. Scope

This protocol applies only to the family support teams and the community mental health teams. A further protocol will be developed for parents with mental health problems in psychiatric hospitals and other specialist units.

3. Background

- On the basis of national statistics it is estimated that approximately 290 Kingston residents will require admission to a psychiatric hospital and about a further 100 will require referral to out patients each year. During 1995–6 the average number of adults receiving help from the three community mental health teams was 904 per quarter – this was a 39% increase on the previous year.
- It has been estimated that approximately 30–40% of adults with mental health problems in Kingston will have children at home. The majority of these parents will be able to provide a good standard of care to their children with the support of their partners and families. However, there is now sound research evidence locally and nationally to show that parental mental health problems are a significant factor threatening the safety and welfare of children.
- Research for the 1997 Kingston Childrens' Services Plan found that parental mental health problems were a significant factor in 26% of cases coming to an Initial Child Protection Conference in 1996–1997.
- National research by Dr Adrian Falkov published in 1996 by the Department of Health looked at fatal child abuse and psychiatric disorder (DOH, 1996). This research found that a third of all cases of fatal child abuse cases he examined had evidence of parental psychiatric disorder, 40% of which was psychosis, 20% depression and 28% personality disorder (including Munchausen Syndrome by Proxy).

- The majority of these parents were natural mothers with sole or main childcare responsibilities.
- In 79% of these cases the children were under 5-years-old, over half had evidence of poor health and developmental problems, two-thirds of them had been subject to child protection cases conferences 85% and had their names placed on the child protection register. Adult mental health services were involved in only 3 out of the 32 cases he reviewed.
- Half the parents concerned had a history of overdose and deliberate self harm and 40% of the parents had contact with psychiatric services in the month prior to the fatal incident. More than one form of mental illness (co-mordity) was a feature in nearly half of the parents and drug dependency was also a significant feature. In two-parent families a significant number of both parents had mental health problems.
- This study highlighted the need for integrated and coordinated services to parents with mental health problems from all the agencies with a responsibility for their health and welfare.
- Studies of young carers have demonstrated the pressures on children of mentally ill parents and the importance of recognizing their needs and providing support.
- Research evidence has shown that women are significantly disadvantaged in their experience of mental health services. Women from ethnic minority groups are likely to experience cumulative disadvantage. It is important that these factors are recognized in the assessment and care management process in a way that does not discriminate against the best interests of the children concerned.
- Children of parents with mental health needs are more likely to be children in need due to their increased risk of health and developmental delay. Inconsistencies and problems in parenting are more likely to mean that they will be children with emotional and behavioural difficulties that will pose further pressures upon their parents. Assisting parents with these problems can be an important part of helping the whole family.
- The research indicates that a significant proportion of parents with serious psychotic mental health problems are a higher risk group for problems in safely parenting their children. However, it is likely that more predominant groups of parents with depressive illness and personality disorders may not attract the same level of priority for mental health services as a parent with a formal mental illness such as paranoid psychosis.

4. Developing the care programme approach

The Care Programme Approach and Care Management Policy between the Council and the Kingston and District NHS Trust sets the framework for an integrated approach to meeting the needs of mentally ill adults in the community in Kingston.

This protocol develops this approach further to provide a framework for the joint assessment of needs of parents with mental health problems by the locality family support teams and the locality community mental health teams.

In many cases mental health services for parents will reduce the risks to the welfare of their children. Similarly, family support services can be an important factor in reducing the stress upon parents with mental health problems.

However, the best interests of children, particularly their safety, must be the paramount consideration for all those concerned.

The community mental health teams are well placed to identify the needs of children of mentally ill parents and to initiate an assessment of their needs through referral to and joint work (where appropriate) with the locality family support teams.

5. Assessment

Social workers in the family support teams and community mental health teams will be pro-active in screening all cases where an adult with mental illness has dependent children, special attention should be given to children under five. The assessment checklist should be used in all cases of parents with mental health problems.

In cases where the parent with primary care responsibilities has a serious mental health problem there should always be a joint assessment carried out by the community mental health team worker and the family support team worker. The decision to combine joint assessment interviews or to conduct them separately will be made by the social workers concerned when the need for a joint assessment has been established.

In complex or difficult cases a joint planning meeting (possibly including a child protection planning meeting) should be held so that a full view of the family's needs can be obtained and a coordinated care plan developed and reviewed.

In cases where the mental health problems have also involved a criminal offence the Probation Service should always be involved in the process and invited to any planning meeting that is arranged for these cases.

In cases where drugs or alcohol are aggravating or complicating factors the community drug and alcohol team should always be involved in the process and invited to any planning meeting that is arranged for these cases. (See protocol for parents with drug or alcohol problems.)

5.1 Joint assessments

Joint assessments may take two forms depending on the circumstances of the case:

A combined joint assessment – this involves community mental health and family support team workers undertaking assessment interviews together at the same time.

A separate joint assessment – this involves these workers undertaking their assessment interviews on different occasions. The assessment information should be shared promptly.

Further action should then be considered which may include a joint planning meeting or a case discussion meeting, a programme of services, referral to other agencies etc. The assessment should consider whether there is a need for co-working and how and when communication will take place.

6. Care management

In cases where there is ongoing work by both the family support team and the community mental health team it will be essential that there is good communication, joint planning and integrated programmes of care for parents with mental health problems that threaten the welfare of their children.

An example of an integrated programme of care is where parental mental health day centre attendance is combined with day care for the children concerned.

Joint care plans must be reviewed on a regular basis. It may be appropriate for community mental health team workers to attend child protection conferences or other meetings where care or protection plans are made. Consultation should always occur between the teams on significant changes in care plans or planned closure of a case.

Where appropriate, family support team social workers should attend care planning meetings or risk assessment meetings held by the community mental health teams or other mental health services.

Local experience has shown that the needs of parents with mental health problems and their children can conflict. This can lead to difficulties in cases held by community mental health teams and family support teams. It is essential that these matters are resolved through joint discussions between the professionals and managers concerned.

7. Working with other agencies

Primary care services such as GPs and health visitors have a key role in supporting parents with mental health problems. They will need to be fully involved in joint assessment and care planning. Consideration should always be given to inviting them to joint planning meetings.

Other services that also should be considered are obstetrics/midwifery, school health services, community paediatrics, Child and Adolescent Psychiatry Service, Educational Welfare Service, Probation Service, schools, police child protection team, WELCARE, homestart, Kingston Women's Aid, housing management and the Homeless Persons unit.

Mental Health groups to consider include MIND, the National Schizophrenia Fellowship, Kingston advocacy services and the Women's Mental Health Project etc.

8. Training

- Social work training has become increasingly specialized so that it can no longer be assumed that all qualified social workers will have some basic experience of mental health and childcare work.
- Childcare awareness training will be provided for all community mental health teams staff and mental health awareness training will be provided for all family support teams staff. All staff will be expected to be able to demonstrate basic awareness in mental health and childcare issues.
- The current training programme includes child protection awareness training for community mental health team staff and this will continue. Joint training will also be provided for the community mental health teams and the family support teams in joint risk assessment and care management for parents with mental health problems.
- A training programme will be developed to introduce the protocol and this will be repeated annually for new staff.

- ASWs should have regular updates on childcare issues as part of their refresher training.
- Induction programmes for new staff in the community mental health teams and family support teams should include familiarization with this protocol.

9. Liaison

Good communication and effective joint working between the community mental health teams and family support teams is essential for an effective service to parents with mental health problems. Team managers from the relevant locality teams should meet on a regular basis to review how the needs of parents with mental health problems are being met, review local working arrangements, consider joint initiatives/ service developments and identify training needs. Joint team meetings or workshops focused on issues of common concern will also help to promote effective joint working.

10. Quality assurance and performance monitoring

- An audit of all community mental health team cases involving parental mental health problems will be conducted in February 1997 by the Performance Review Section.
- A sample of all S.47 and safeguarding assessment cases where parental mental health problems are a feature will be reviewed regularly in the Case Monitoring sub group of the Area Child Protection Committee.
- An annual review of the protocol will be conducted by the Principal Manager Family Support and Child Protection, Principal Manager Mental Health, and other relevant senior health service managers and professionals.
- Performance indicators will be developed by the Performance Review Section to monitor the operation of the protocol.

Guidance notes for the protocol

Overview

All mental health referrals/cases involving parents or carers will be screened by the community mental health teams. The priority allocated to each case and the corresponding response to any identified concerns or needs will depend on the circumstances of each case and will fall into one of four categories.

Similarly, the children and families family support teams will screen all referrals/ cases for any identified parental mental concerns or needs. The priority allocated to each case and the corresponding response will also fall into one of four categories.

See the protocol flow chart.

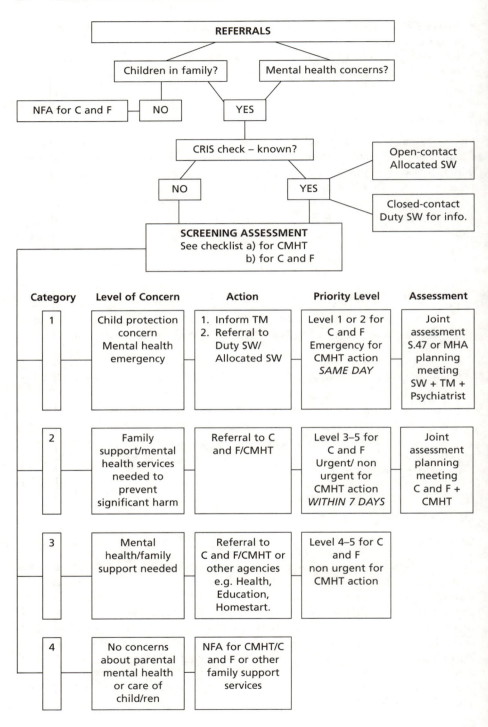

Category 1

High level – child protection concerns and/or urgent mental health concerns

This category covers explicit child protection concerns and/or a mental health emergency. The community mental health teams or family support team social workers will be responsible for identifying these cases using the assessment checklists.

All child protection or urgent mental health concerns identified will be referred to children and families services or community mental health teams immediately and will lead to a joint planning meeting. This will also incorporate the requirements of a S.47 Planning Meeting.

If a Mental Health Act assessment is also indicated then this should also be planned at this joint meeting unless there are good reasons for not doing so.

Category 2

Mental health services and/or family support required to prevent significant harm to individuals or families

This covers:

Concerns for the care or treatment of children which do not require an urgent child protection response but do require a safeguarding response or promotional services. These cases can include concerns about quality of care, e.g. increasing neglect, relationship problems, the risk of family breakdown leading to a hospital admission and/or for a child to be 'looked after'.

Concerns for parental mental health that do not require an urgent ASW assessment or urgent mental health intervention but do require support, e.g. when a significant deterioration in parental mental health has occurred.

The need for a joint planning meeting for a joint assessment should be considered. The format of joint assessment should be agreed at the point of referral or at the joint planning meeting.

Category 3

Family support or mental health services needed to promote the welfare of individuals and families

This category covers family support or mental health needs that do not indicate a risk of significant harm to the children concerned or a risk of a significant mental health problem.

This category applies to parents with mental health problems who can be supported through promotional mental health or family support services (such as day care sponsorship) or by voluntary and universal statutory services, e.g. GPs, HVs, MIND, counselling services, Relate etc.

Category 4

Mental health or family support services not required

This category covers parents with mental health problems who are able to cope and meet the needs of their children with support from family and friends in the community. There will be no significant concerns for the mental health of the parent or the welfare of children and no need for referral for assessment or services from mental health or family support agencies.

Crossing over between services: the Lewisham experience

Marie Diggins

Lewisham is an inner city multicultural London borough. Along with other inner London boroughs, Lewisham has a higher than average incidence of mental illness. The inner city environment, its low socio-economic status and high levels of unemployment lead to a heavy overuse of psychiatric in-patient services, with bed occupancy rates of more than 100 per cent. Rates of formal admissions under the Mental Health Act 1983 (Department of Health, 1983) and use of secure and medium secure beds are well above the national average.

Since 1992, following the introduction of the Children Act 1989 (Department of Health, 1989) and the Community Care Act 1990 (Department of Health, 1990b), Lewisham Social Services has undergone a series of reorganizations. Most noticeable to social work practitioners has been the move away from generic work in favour of specialisms and the dividing of services into the 'purchaser and provider' split.

Specialization versus genericism

I qualified as a social worker in 1989 when one of the 'buzz' words of the time was the importance of taking a 'holistic' approach when assessing or working with individuals and families. The move to specialisms has forced the focus of some of our work to be identified now as either 'adult centred' or 'child centred'.

Looking back to my experience of generic work, many social workers within teams had specific interests or expertise that led to them 'semi-specializing' in certain areas, although duty social work offered a broader experience.

It has been argued both ways; that generic social work was too broad, practitioners were frustrated at being 'Jack of all trades, master of none!', and sufficient expertise in any one area could not be achieved. A contrary argument is that in specializing in one area, a wider systemic perspective cannot be maintained to view problems in context so easily.

Specialisms are here to stay, at least for some time, therefore, the question of favouring either approach will not be investigated or discussed further here.

In order that specialist approaches do not inhibit a holistic assessment of individuals and families, there is an expectation in the department, and inherent in national and local policy, that information and cooperation will flow between those involved, and that joint planning and working together will take place between agencies and with families. Although this expectation is paramount and logical, to expect the best outcomes, in practice this does not always go smoothly. Furthermore, families may have a number of other professionals besides social workers involved, i.e. a psychiatrist and CPNs for the parents. These workers will be 'adult centred' and therefore will not necessarily pick up on children's issues and many would not see this as their responsibility.

Studies and inquiry reports have shown that when working with families where the parent has a mental health problem, it can be all too easy for intervention to be very 'adult focused', making it difficult to prioritize children's needs or the needs of the adults as parents (Falkov, 1995; Woodley Inquiry Team, 1995).

The whole topic of public services involvement with these families has proved to be of national and, certainly in Lewisham, of local interest over the last 2 years. Many authorities and organizations are trying to address these issues that have arisen from their contact and work with families in need.

The process of moving from being a generic social worker to a specialist social worker, whether it be in childcare or mental health, is difficult to describe. It was for many a matter of changing into a specialist social worker overnight.

Strangely and very quickly, however, the commonalities that social workers had shared previously, for example the ability to carry out comprehensive assessments with various service-user groups, were quick to dwindle. Unwritten and unspoken demarcations and barriers became apparent.

Previously, in generic teams, any specialist knowledge or skills workers may have developed from their experience or training, was always over and above their general duties; they were social workers first, and experts second. They were social workers first and foremost and as such with management support were required to work with all groups of people. They would be able to carry out a comprehensive holistic assessment and when necessary other professional expertise was called in if and when necessary, i.e. medical and legal opinions.

What seemed and seems to have happened in Lewisham and other local authorities is that social workers have reported feeling quickly deskilled in working with user groups outside their own specialism. When questioned further this deskilling process extends, it seems, to not recognizing or feeling confident in using transferable skills. So does this now mean expert first and social worker second!

By separating the specialisms, i.e. mental health and childcare, this seems to have imposed or allowed people to create unhelpful demarcations that do not allow peoples' roles as parents and their children to be given the attention they deserve, whereas the introduction of specialization was meant to contribute additional expertise to the social work services people were receiving.

It is not all a picture of doom and gloom and Lewisham like many other local authorities has recognized the difficulties very quickly. As part of the whole process of developing specialisms and working together, Lewisham are taking steps to try to carefully move towards a more equitable and comprehensive approach to the difficulties that many of these families face.

The following text aims to look at some related initiatives in Lewisham that attempt to recognize the needs of the adult as a parent and the needs of the child in ways that are not mutually exclusive of each other, and where social services are taking the lead in being proactive in really getting to grips with effective 'working together' to meet the needs of this service user group.

Adventure weekends

Public and professional attention has recently focused on the dilemmas and isolation of young carers and the difficulties in identifying who and where they are and how to meet their needs (Elliott, 1992; Deardon and Becker, 1995). The focus on this particular group has increased with the introduction of the Children Act 1989 (Department of Health, 1989) and the Community Care Act 1990 (Department of Health, 1990b) and more recently with the Carers Services and Recognition Act 1996 (Department of Health, 1996c). The Adventure Weekend Breaks Project described below, and the other initiatives mentioned in this chapter, are concerned with all children in these families, not only young carers. Those caring for a mentally ill parent may not necessarily see themselves as young carers and highlighting this group can diminish in some children's eyes what they actually do.

Research suggests that when children are used to coping with so much, they appear capable and stable, giving no indication of the bewilderment they feel inside themselves. Some do not even have the vocabulary to describe what is happening and they might think why would anyone want to know anyway? (MIND, 1996).

One study reveals that children caring for a mentally ill parent have less obvious but more complicated needs than those whose parents have visible, predictable illnesses or disabilities (Elliott, 1992) Some doctors, guarding the confidentiality of the patients, refuse to discuss the illness with the family or take its wider implications on board. Some teachers do not think to find out if there is a reason other than carelessness for a child being routinely late for school or not handing in homework. 'Information is vitally important in every aspect of working with these children, there are hundreds of children all over the country wondering if their parent is "mad" or going to die because they keep saying they want to, but have no way of finding out what is going on and why. Their voices, stifled by the ignorance and stigma still surrounding mental distress, must be heard before many more of them are robbed of their youth' (MIND, 1996).

The Adventure Weekend Breaks were initiated for a variety of reasons:

- To provide respite opportunities for parents and their children.
- To offer the children a chance to enjoy a weekend of fun and adventure in the company of others who may share similar experiences.
- To offer the parents a chance to spend some time without childcare responsibilities in the knowledge that their child would be well looked after.
- For social workers from both specialisms (mental health and childcare) to spend a significant amount of time directly working with the children and each other.

– For these social workers to take back to their own teams their experiences and to promote the needs of children in these families.
– For social workers to refresh or improve their skills in communicating with children.

This project was highly successful and won a Community Care Enterprise Award in 1995. It is a very simple initiative that offers a direct service to young people and their parents and enables staff to consider the wider needs of these families and of joint working.

As a result of the success of this project the social workers involved decided to try to take things forward and try to identify and initiate the development of tackling the crossover issues and to provide more hands-on support services.

'Partnership or polarization?'

The question I set myself in designing the following research project was 'How can Lewisham Social Services Department help to facilitate effective joint agency and intra-agency work with families where the parents have mental health problems?'

The aim of the study

To influence social work practice in Lewisham Social Services Department to enable children's needs to be viewed as a priority and addressed in families where either parent has a mental health problem.

Objectives to meet this aim

To find out the views of social work managers and staff in Lewisham and to compare these views with findings from other research and in relation to legislation.

Method

The study focused on the collection of both qualitative and quantitative material and the method used is known as 'Triangulation'. Cheetham *et al.* (1994, p. 47) describe this as:

> 'Triangulation of method in which several different methods of data collection are employed in a single study provides a means of validating information derived from different sources and permits the weaknesses and strengths of different data collection methods to be balanced.'

The research was carried out in four parts.

A questionnaire

To social workers working in the areas of childcare or mental health/adult teams. A cross-section of workers was needed as there is no 'typical' social work role with these families.

A conference on childcare and adult mental health

Using the findings from workshops that were organized as part of a mini-conference looking at childcare and adult mental health. Questionnaires were also completed at the conference.

Individual interviews

A series of individual semi-structured interviews carried out with a cross-section of service unit managers from the children and family social work teams and from the adult/mental health teams.

Group interview

A semi-structured group interview with the director of Lewisham social services, the assistant director for purchasing services and the assistant director from the provider side.

I chose to concentrate on four areas within the London Borough of Lewisham Social Services Department and to compare my findings with existing information and literature as outlined above. The four areas are:

- Social work skills.
- Working together – within the agency and with other agencies.
- Training.
- Resources.

Summary of the main findings and recommendations

Power and stereotypes are both key components of discrimination and oppression, therefore their impact on service users and systems of service delivery must be scrutinized and monitored if the department's commitment to anti-discriminatory practice is to be meaningful. Criteria for the delivery of a service should not depend on whether the relationship between key managers is 'good' or 'bad', nor should people be sent back and forth if a label of 'mental illness' or 'child abuse' has or has not been discovered.

The preoccupation of who has overall responsibility for a case, or budgetary responsibility, has been an issue for members of the department. Findings also show that there is an opinion that a major priority for some is to shift any work or responsibility elsewhere if possible. Additionally a response from every sector of the departmental hierarchy was that the type of service a service user receives depends to a certain extent on how the respective managers 'get on' in the various districts. For some this situation was blamed on the absence of guidelines. If this is not addressed it can only have a deleterious and discriminatory effect on service users and does not represent an equitable approach to service delivery. The resources wasted in social workers' time doing this can only put a further drain on what is available and ultimately have a detrimental effect on the user.

At the time of the study the situation could be likened to the analogy of the 'chicken and egg', i.e. which came first? the chicken or the egg? If a parent who suffers with severe mental health problems needs some childcare support, who will respond? Will it be the childcare team because it is a difficulty with parenting,? Will it be the adult team because the parent has a mental health problem? Will it be both or neither because a decision cannot be made? All of these scenarios seem possible within the system with its inbuilt arbitrariness.

Skills

The findings showed some discrepancy across the department in relation to why workers were feeling so deskilled, and what might be done to remedy that. Everyone seemed in agreement that social workers should ideally be able to assess family situations to a degree where they could identify mental health and childcare concerns whatever their specialism. However, the findings taken literally show that respondents' opinions of what skills should exist does not seem to be the case at the moment. Workers and managers made a variety of suggestions as to how this might be remedied. Some ideas contradicted each other. For example, workers wanted accountability for cases to be clearer but they also wanted more cases to be jointly allocated between the teams, whilst the department wanted to see one worker or team taking overall case responsibility.

Recommendations

- The designation of one senior social worker in each children and family team and in each sector of the new mental health social work teams to be trained and involved in both mental health and childcare, with the aim of increasing the teams' skills through the dissemination of knowledge and experience via the duty system, supervision and liaison with other teams.
- A comprehensive joint and multi-agency training strategy – see under 'Training' recommendations.
- Monitoring of skills and training needs via the existing Employee Development Scheme and supervision.
- Risk assessment checklists highlighting combined risk factors.
- Pre-determined checklists for multidisciplinary case management – see 'Working together' recommendations.
- Up-to-date resource information useful to both specialisms.

Working together

The responses received were heavily weighted towards issues relating to joint working within the department. Responses received in relation to working with other agencies were minimal in comparison. Two managers suggested 'let us get our own house in order first'.

Important barriers to collaboration seem to be:

- Misunderstanding of each other's roles.
- Stereotyping.
- Different agendas and priorities.

- Different status.
- Workload fears.
- Inadequate information.
- Agency and management constraints, e.g. budgets.

People seem unclear of each other's roles, and their own at times, in relation to who does what in casework or care management. There was a substantial body of feeling from adult workers that they were not respected by their children and family counterparts. They felt that childcare workers peddled a view that it is less prestigious and not so difficult a job to be a mental health/adult social worker as it is to be a childcare social worker.

The use of stereotyping in order to fit cases to certain teams or resources is apparent, as are the difficulties in coming to grips with the different philosophies and agendas used by each specialist team. Workload fears were illustrated 'that if work can be referred elsewhere this should be a priority'. The notion that childcare teams do not have enough social workers and are not so well resourced in comparison with adult teams, was given as a reason by adult workers and some managers for the perceived reluctance by children and family teams to engage in joint working. Information sharing and communication seemed to many to happen in an *ad hoc* way and there was an overall sense that each team did not know what the current developments were in their corresponding team or specialism. This may account for the rise of generalizations and false beliefs.

Many workers, particularly children and family workers, expressed the opinion that managers should be taking more of a lead in facilitating joint working and should show more commitment to this. They would like to see regular joint meetings about difficult cases and plans to strengthen collaboration between locality teams.

Recommendations

- For a designated member of the department to be given the responsibility for developing, facilitating and monitoring a joint intra- and inter-agency strategy to working specifically with these two combined service-user groups.
- To share and increase the circulation of information about the structures and procedures of each group through training, written information and liaison between teams.
- The designation of one senior social worker post in each team to act as a specialist worker in both childcare and mental health (see 'Skills' recommendations above) to oversee their tasks in relation to working together. They would also act as liaison between teams on difficult cases, to look at more imaginative and cost-effective ways of joint funding between teams and to act as representatives at key departmental meetings.
- For the department to take the lead in encouraging other key agencies, perhaps via the Area Child Protection Committee, to appoint key liaison workers to work together using a locality model on local projects or meetings on specified topics specifically relating to these families and joint working.

- For regular and reliable recording of the at-risk population by creating adaptations to existing forms in adult mental health and childcare, incorporating this where possible with the social services information database.
- The development of multi-agency forms for assessment, care management and after-care plans and joint agency plans for crisis intervention, to provide clarification and checklists for workers and easier dissemination of information.
- A need for senior management support in formalizing a strategy and in helping to re-assess the criteria for resources including social work allocation in teams, by re-formulating the criteria to include the combined risks these families may present and to acknowledge and give permission for the shift towards preventative work to take place.

Training

The overall opinion from respondents was that workers on the whole were feeling deskilled or did not have the all-round experience of assessing adult mental health and childcare together. Newly qualified workers, who are more apparent in children and families teams, may have fairly up-to-date knowledge but no firm grounding in practice. The department and a minority of other respondents also suggested that the skills have not been lost, rather that people have lost confidence in areas they are not practising in regularly and that many skills, particularly in assessment, are transferable and it is 'social workers first, specialists second'.

It was generally agreed that ongoing refresher training should be available to both teams, with more intensive training for senior social workers and supervisors as discussed in 'Skills' above.

Everybody seemed in agreement that joint training and multidisciplinary training was the preferred option in as many cases as possible. However, it was expressed that because of the differing skills in each other's specialist areas it might be difficult to design and carry out joint training that would meet everyone's needs.

Recommendations

- For a specific training strategy to be included in the department's training plan, and for ongoing refresher training that takes into account the varying needs in teams that specifically address the joint issues arising from the two specialisms.
- To utilize the existing expertise in the department by encouraging members of the department to take part in organizing and facilitating training.
- To encourage user participation where possible in the planning and delivery of training.
- To prioritize training needs for those acting as the designated liaison senior social workers, if this is agreed.
- To liaise with the provider side of the department to ensure that any possible sharing of training materials and packages takes place.
- Prioritizing anti-discriminatory practice specifically in relation to mental illness and working with children in all aspects of any training package.
- In order to aid clarification of roles, to aim to deliver as much training as possible in an inter- or intra-agency way.

Resources

The following shows the type of resources respondents want to see more of:

- Family support services – practical support by staff trained in mental health and childcare.
- Twenty-four-hour crisis intervention.
- Respite opportunities for parent and child.
- Direct work with children, i.e. groupwork.
- Befrienders.
- Specialist foster care.
- Specialist 'contact' facilities for those children 'looked after' by the local authority.
- A multidisciplinary family assessment resource that includes adult and child psychiatric input.

The department is in the process of planning with other agencies the development of further family support services, mental health day-care for black service users and a specialist team that will support people in their own homes. With the development of the new mental health team there will also be new posts for additional hospital, forensic and rehabilitation social workers.

During the discussion within the department it was clear that there are already moves being made towards bringing together the two sides of the in-house provider units, i.e. childcare and adult mental health. By doing this the aim is to try to bridge the gap that exists and to open up services to accommodate these families in a much more constructive way, by tackling the discrimination that exists in current provision whereby mental health service users are excluded from adult services if they are parents because there are no childcare facilities, and in childcare where the severity of the parent's illness can preclude children and parents benefiting from childcare services because there are not the resources to cope with the presenting difficulties.

Recommendations

- Training to be given in provider locations on crossover issues.
- As outlined by the departments, possible secondments between workers in childcare provider services and mental health provider services to encourage greater liaison and identification on how services might be able to 'crossover'.
- For locality meetings – described above – to target what they need specifically from services and then to negotiate contracts and use of budgets to provide more imaginative packages of care, i.e. if several people are needing help with parenting skills across teams it may be more beneficial and cost effective to offer a parenting skills group run by family care workers than to allocate a worker to each family.

Research summary and conclusion

Throughout the study process there was a willingness across Lewisham Social Services Department to identify areas for improvement and change, with the longer term aim of benefiting the families that are the focus for the research. People's honesty about their views and experiences greatly aided the process, especially in clarifying what are assumptions and what is actually happening in the department.

As the focus of the study is on identifying areas for change, it inevitably tends to record more situations where the department may be wanting to improve service delivery, rather than where things are working well. The development of the new specialist mental health team due to be in operation in June 1997 provides the timely opportunity for some of the issues raised here to be incorporated into the planning of this new team. It is envisaged that the new team will have much closer links with adult psychiatric services, which may create, amongst other opportunities, the possibility of earlier comprehensive multi-disciplinary assessments for families.

It would be impossible for the department to come up with a strategy or plans to cover all eventualities or satisfy every training need. In my recommendations, I have tried to evaluate the research responses against the background of the literature and legislation, in order to formulate ideas that may be used individually or in their entirety. Knowing that resourcing new or different ideas can be costly, I have tried to recommend suggestions that relate more to the re-focusing of existing resources, or utilizing more effectively expertise already in existence.

The most overriding need, both for the department and service users, is the validation of the importance that the department places on these issues, by designating someone to coordinate, develop and monitor the process of effective working together with the ultimate aim of offering services that are wanted by service users.

As a practitioner/researcher, having had the opportunity of talking to many members of the department and gathering personal and professional views, I appreciated the amount of transferable knowledge and skills that exists in the department and the opportunities available for that to be utilized to a greater degree in the four areas used above: skills, working together, training and resources, in order to move the goal of improved working practices and service delivery onwards. This leads onto the third and final initiative.

FamilyBridge

The final example chosen from Lewisham's initiatives is one that has developed alongside the research process above, and originated from the efforts of the social workers who began with the modest Adventure Weekend project. Throughout the research process other agencies and individuals with an interest and commitment to promoting better working together with and for these families met, at the invitation of social services, to form a group that would concentrate on promoting the interests of these families with the ultimate aim of improving service delivery to them and initiating new services.

The lead agencies have been Lewisham Social Services, the Guy's Lewisham Mental Health Trust, the Family Welfare Association, Lewisham Users Forum and the Lewisham Area Child Protection Committee.

The group was further inspired by a conference held early in 1997 entitled 'Crossover Issues' which was organized by the Lewisham ACPC and attended by a variety of agencies and service users.

The project has managed to obtain funding now for the development of the multi-agency 'FamilyBridge' which will be an umbrella resource that incorporates a variety of provider services alongside a focus of developing multi-agency training, policy, publications, and research and evaluation. The FamilyBridge aims to bring together the above initiatives and others in Lewisham that are concerned with these families. I worked with Amy Weir to develop a bid to the Department of Health and 3 years' funding for the project was awarded.

Postscript (Janet's story)

The following is some prose written by one of my own social work clients, Janet. Janet grew up with a mother who suffered with manic depression and Janet's childhood was severely disrupted by this. Janet coped the best she could in the circumstances. She developed some ingenious and sometimes shocking defence mechanisms that enabled her to cope with the abandonment and loss she felt.

As a young adult, Janet developed manic depression and for many years has suffered with severe and enduring mental illness. She has a son of her own who is in his 20s and Janet cannot help but worry about him and what she considers might be the effects of her own illness on him. There is also the niggling worry – 'what if he develops the same illness? After all, it has run in two generations so far!'

Janet manages her life remarkably well and is a survivor of the mental health system and the many things life has thrown at her. One of her many ambitions is to record some of her life experiences on paper. My impression is that she is considerably gifted in portraying very human and thought-provoking material. It is having the privilege of working with Janet and others that has taught me so much in my social work career and has given me the inspiration and energy to carry out this piece of work. Without further ado, here is Janet's prose, which she has called *Taking Care*.

Taking Care

I suppose my mother failed me, but then, I failed her. I wasn't a good minder, not like the ones you read about in the paper. 'Little angel cares unaided as Mother lies in coma' . . . Susie (6) took wing to the kitchen and fetched her Mother the life-support spoonful of sugar. Mother Julie (24) of one-parent family, said, 'she's great – more of a friend than a daughter'. I, on the other hand, began a lifetime's work going from inadequate child to sick parent. First, aged 13, I stopped listening to Mother about 'How-to-cope-in-an-Emergency' and became one. I refused to go to school. I fell off the bus that would take me there and into the bed I should have left.

That way, I got a lot of care. Sometimes I was noticed too much, and they started to coax me out of my hibernation, but at least it was better than my Mum being ill on me. Was she ill then, or was I the focus of everyone's attention? I can't remember, but I do know that a child cannot manipulate adults completely – adults are bigger after all and they have certain powers.

The care plan now was to get me to boarding school, away from it all (they meant my Mum), so I could learn to stand on my own two feet (there was nothing wrong with them. It was my heart that hurt). Still, after 5 years there, I began to level. Failed 11+, but got 2 Os and an A. When I wasn't behaving like a child, I started to grow up.

Time to move on – who better than a problem child to teach children? College came – and went, as I discovered trying to read a library of teachers' literature. I went to sick bay, then hospital to ward off disaster. But life overwhelmed me, and like my mother, I let my pain loose. Eventually, they let me leave to clean up for old ladies like my Granny.

I got engaged and disentangled before I married someone else. We had a baby and I sat him in my lap for 'Listen with Mother'. I was happy then, too happy, before I fell off the top and couldn't get up. That's how it went from there and my son had to go with it, but not fall off himself. I was not at the school gate to meet him. Aunties took my place. He came to see me, through high gates and down long corridors. Sometimes, I did not pick him up. In the ward next door, he had Hospital Tea with his Granny. Perched high on cushions, he ate his boiled egg and soldiers, keeping his eye on his place with Granny.

At 11, he went to Secondary School. He was bullied there and emotionally bruised at home. The Authorities thought he should have a chance to stand on his own two feet – did they ache as much as my heart at his enthusiasm? He went to boarding school and learned to live again. He discovered that whereas before he had only one person's unpredictable behaviour to manage, now there were 11 in his Dorm . . .

I watched him settle down gradually, then gatecrashed his GCSEs by leaving his father. (Do the political goings-on of 1890 in a History paper mean much to a 16-year-old trapped in 1990?)

It is now 1996 and I have been 'newly-wed' for nearly 4 years. I do not have a new mind to go with my present husband, but maybe there is hope through his refusal to give up on me. My son, with his big feet, and even larger heart, has said he bears me no ill will. Perhaps he has come some way to a compromise. He has not broken the birth cord, but neither has he let it strangle him.

(Janet Joyce, 1996)

I would like to conclude this chapter by including one more piece of prose by Janet.

Careless

When I was two or three, my Mother gathered me onto her lap for 'Listen with Mother' on the wireless. I treasure that memory of being a child with an adult, but later the programme changed.

First it was 'Go and see Mother' down endless corridors to a starched bed too high for me to perch on. Next, it was 'Hear your Mother crying and screaming her unhappiness out loud'. I stared at my mat and ate my boiled egg like a soldier.

One night, she left. No more noise, just emptiness, which was worse. But I got her back, courtesy of the Courts, and she was my Mum again. It didn't last. That morning, my Mum, my little sister and I were together for breakfast. It was a tiny flat, and we ate scrambled eggs. I think my Mum cooked it – that's another thing Mothers are for. She went upstairs and I felt funny. I got my sister to help with the washing up. Someone's hands were holding the tea-towel when Mum came downstairs again. She was getting into a coat. I froze. 'You'll have to let yourselves out today, girls. I'm going to Bexley Hospital. Lock up and go to school. After school, go to Granny'.

Of course we did all that. It was 'Listen to Mother'. I knew the rules and I loved my Granny. But Mothers don't just leave their children. When mine did, she left me with a re-severed cord and an insatiable thirst for emotional blood transfusions.   (Janet Joyce, 1996)

Finally, the questionnaire set out in full below was sent to social workers who participated in my research project.

Partnership or polarization? Childcare and adult mental health research

The attached questionnaire forms part of a research process currently being carried out in Lewisham. The research is concerned with social work with families where either parent has a mental health problem.

The questionnaire consists of a variety of questions under the following category headings:

– Social work skills
– Working together – intra/specializations
– Miscellaneous

The questionnaire is being sent to social workers in both adult and children and family teams and therefore some questions will seem more relevant than others depending on which team you come from. Please try and complete all of the questions – there are not necessarily any right or wrong answers and the forms will remain anonymous. If you do not or cannot answer a question please indicate why.

It takes roughly 20 minutes to fill in this questionnaire and your comments will form the bulk of the research data which in turn will be translated into conclusions and recommendations that will be presented to the directorate, therefore, this is a real opportunity to put forward your views.

Please remember when answering the questions that all questions refer to only those families where the parent/parents have a mental health problem and should be answered keeping that in mind.

Thank you for agreeing to complete this questionnaire. A report of the research findings will be available to teams at the end of the year.

Please complete the following details before starting the questionnaire

Do you work for an adult team?	YES/NO
Are you a mental health specialist?	YES/NO
Do you work in a children and family team?	YES/NO
What grade are you? (e.g. basic grade, senior, manager)	....
Have you worked as a generic social worker?	YES/NO
Do you have experience of childcare work?	YES/NO
Do you have experience of mental health work?	YES/NO

SOCIAL WORK SKILLS

(1) What do you think are the main issues that have arisen for mental health social workers in Lewisham since 1992 in working with these families?

....
....
....
....

(2) What do you think are the main issues that have arisen for children and family social workers in Lewisham since 1992 in working with these families?

....
....
....
....

(3) What range of skills do mental health social workers need in childcare and child protection?

....
....
....
....

(4) In your opinion are Lewisham adult/mental health social workers skilled enough in the areas you have identified   YES/NO

....
....
....
....

(5) What range of skills do children and family social workers need in mental health?

....
....
....
....

(6) In your opinion are Lewisham children and family social workers skilled enough in the areas you have identified   YES/NO. If yes, how?

....

....

....

....

(7) Given that social workers in Lewisham all work in specialist teams do workers achieve and maintain these skills and experience?   YES/NO. If yes, how?

....

....

....

....

(8) Has your team officially identified team members who have a specialist interest or expertise in working with these families   YES/NO

(9) Do you agree with the following statement – All senior social workers should be trained and have ongoing practice experience in both mental health and childcare?   YES/NO

(10) Do you think the 'Care Programme Approach' has benefited those people with mental health problems who are parents?   YES/NO

(11) Much that has been written over the last few years suggests that there are many children in families whose needs are hidden because of the adult and child's inability or fear of approaching agencies for help. If you agree with this statement, how can we begin to identify these children that are 'hidden' either through our own agency or working with other agencies?

....

....

....

....

(12) Would you agree that during assessments (health or other) of all those coming into the psychiatric system, some part of the assessment should focus on whether there are any parenting difficulties as a direct or indirect result of the parents' mental health problems. Should the focus be on identifying needs of both parent and child?

YES/NO

WORKING TOGETHER – INTRA/SPECIALIZATIONS

(13) What is your perception and experience of joint working between the children and adult social work teams with these families?   POOR/AVERAGE/GOOD

(14) What are the issues regarding joint working for the managers? and workers?

....

....

....

(15) Given the Care Programme Approach and the necessity for childcare or child protection plans for those families already known to the department is the amount of information incorporated into an overall plan?   YES/NO

(16) In jointly held cases would an agreement outlining the following roles and responsibilities be helpful? If yes, please tick those you feel important to include
   (a) Are managers jointly managing the case?
   (b) How is supervision to be arranged for the overall case?
   (c) Do workers have access to appropriate specialist consultation when needed?
   (d) Are the case notes to be combined?
   (e) Requirements for attendance at multidisciplinary meetings?
   (f) Identified budgets for purchasing resources?
   (g) Childcare coordinator role?
   (h) Anything else?
   ....
   ....
   ....

(17) Has the move for workers into specializations helped or hindered families that have two workers involved, i.e. a children and families social worker and a mental health social worker?   YES/NO
   ....
   ....
   ....
   ....

(18) What lessons have been learnt since the introductions of specialisms in relation to working jointly with these families?
   ....
   ....
   ....
   ....

(19) Do mental health resources in Lewisham take into account the needs of those who are parents with young children?   YES/NO

(20) Are you aware of any written guidelines or policy within the department relating to working jointly with these families? If YES can you say what this is?
   ....
   ....
   ....
   ....

(21) Do you or your team follow any guidance?   YES/NO. If yes, what?
   ....
   ....
   ....
   ....

WORKING TOGETHER – INTER-AGENCY

(22) In cases you are aware of, which of the following health professionals are invited to childcare conferences or planning meetings and do they attend?

	INVITED	ATTENDANCE
G.P	YES/NO	poor/average/good
Adult Psychiatrist	YES/NO	poor/average/good
Child Psychiatrist	YES/NO	poor/average/good
Community Psychiatric Nurse	YES/NO	poor/average/good
Adult Team Social Worker	YES/NO	poor/average/good

(23) Are there any problems regarding access to medical information or consultation regarding the parents' mental health problems and the possible effects of their mental health on their children and their parenting ability?　　　　YES/NO

(24) When a Child Protection issue is identified do all professionals in the multidisciplinary system understand their roles and responsibilities and those of others in relation to the child?　　　　YES/NO

(25) If workers are described as either 'adult'- or 'child'-centred/focused how well do we in Lewisham ensure that the child's needs remain paramount?
Please tick on a scale of 1 to 10:
very poor　1　2　3　4　5　6　7　8　9　10　very good

MISCELLANEOUS

(26) Would you like to see more joint training opportunities particularly in relation to crossover issues in working with these families?　　　　YES/NO

(27) Which of the following areas would you like to see included in joint training?
(a) Risk assessment　　　　YES/NO
(b) Clarification of professionals' roles　　　　YES/NO
(c) Policy issues　　　　YES/NO
(d) Crisis intervention for the family　　　　YES/NO
(e) Parenting skills　　　　YES/NO
(f) Effects on children of parental mental health　　　　YES/NO
(g) Legal framework　　　　YES/NO
(h) Effective joint working strategies　　　　YES/NO
(i) Anything else?
....
....
....

(28) 'The provision of community care services should ensure that young carers are not expected to carry inappropriate levels of caring responsibilities. It should not be assumed that children should take on similar levels of caring responsibilities to adults'. Following the introduction of the Carers Recognition and Services Act Lewisham guidelines on implementation advise that Young Carers Core

Assessment of Needs should be carried out by adult team workers. How many assessments of this kind have you been involved in or have you referred?

....

....

....

....

(29) Have you any comments about the current Community Care Carers Assessment form that is used and its suitability for young carers?

....

....

....

....

If you have <u>not</u> seen or used one of these forms please indicate   YES/NO

(30) Please tick which of the following resources you would like to see available for these families?
   (a) Family support services – with staff trained in mental health and childcare
   (b) Twenty-four-hour crisis support
   (c) Respite care opportunities for parent and child
   (d) Direct work with children, i.e. groupwork, befrienders, specialist foster care
   (e) A multidisciplinary family assessment resource providing comprehensive assessments and recommendations for complex and time-consuming cases?
   (f) Specialist 'contact' arrangements for those children 'looked after'?
   (g) Anything else?

....

....

....

(31) Black people are over-represented in the mental health system and black women with mental health problems are far more likely to have their children received into care. Alongside this the emphasis of the Care Programme Approach is to provide for those people in the system who are most disadvantaged and specifically black people with mental health problems. How can we provide equal opportunity to services for this group in Lewisham to begin to redress these issues?

....

....

....

....

(32) Lewisham will soon see the opening of a new black mental health centre. How would you like to see the centre provide for people with children?

....

....

....

....

Please add any other comments you may have. If you feel this questionnaire has not provided you with the opportunity to express particular points that you feel are relevant or you would like to contribute further to the research process, please indicate this by adding your name and contact number at the end of this questionnaire, alternatively you can contact Marie Diggins directly at the Northover Mental Health Centre on 0181–461–5577, where it will be possible to arrange an individual interview.

Thank you very much for completing this questionnaire. A report of the research findings will be available to social work teams at the end of 1996.

The contribution of the voluntary sector to innovation and development

Christopher P. Hanvey

Introductory comments by Amy Weir

The voluntary sector has been involved in a variety of different projects and campaigns over the last few years to support families and children affected by mental illness.

MIND in particular has been involved in trying to highlight the need to cater specifically for the needs of women with mental health problems and their children. In 1994, they ran a campaign called 'Breakthrough' in support of the needs of women. Women are still more likely than men to be admitted to psychiatric hospitals. MIND has drawn attention to the inadequacy of the services available to these women and their children. There is still a lack of facilities for children to visit their parents in hospital. Crèche arrangements within outpatient departments are also extremely rare.

The Association for Postnatal Illness runs a volunteer register across the country for women who find it difficult to cope with their children and who are suffering from postnatal illness. Other organizations – like the New Parent Infant Network (NEWPIN) – have set up support groups to help mothers with depression.

Other organizations – such as Barnardos – have been involved in seeking to support and meet the needs of children affected by their parent's mental illness. For instance, a 3-year pilot support and befriending scheme was established in Leeds by Barnardos with financial support from Leeds City Council. The project has operated with volunteers who have organized outings as well as giving practical and emotional support.

At the Family Welfare Association (FWA) I developed innovative services to meet the needs of families in Lambeth and Lewisham with financial support from the Department of Health. The first project in Lambeth sought to try to understand what services would enable families to be effectively supported with the care of their children. The Lewisham project, run by the FWA, is to set up a family resource centre dedicated to meeting the needs of families affected by mental illness – this is to be known as FamilyBridge (see Chapter 12).

The NSPCC has been involved in a major project in Brent to consider what service approach is most likely to fit with the needs of local families. Having reviewed the current state of knowledge about these issues, local focus groups of service users were established to seek views about the services required. A multi-agency steering group of the ACPC in Brent is directing a strategy to improve practice and to respond to the views of service users. The families interviewed were enthusiastic about the research. All the families felt strongly that better services would make a difference to their quality of life, and would help them to deal with the painful experiences of living with mental illness.

What follows is a more detailed description by Dr Chris Hanvey about the work of a contact centre at the Thomas Coram Foundation, a national voluntary organization, in London.

How the voluntary sector can make a difference

Samuel Johnson was the source of many apocryphal stories. One such concerned his questioning, by a friend, as to why his dictionary had defined 'pastern' as the knee, rather than the foot, of a horse. 'Ignorance, madam, pure ignorance' was the robust and characteristic reply. Such a response might be equally applicable to the question as to why health and social services agencies rarely make a link between mental health and child protection. Where, for example, are the national statistics on the number of children on child protection registers, where one or both carers have some form of mental illness? Or conversely, do we really know if a correlation exists between severe mental health problems and the incidence of child abuse?

One analogy is with alcohol services. Raising awareness, within a welfare agency, of the prevalence of alcohol abuse can lead to a greater openness in recognizing alcohol problems in clinics and on individual caseloads. A similar willingness to place mental health and child protection issues together should assist in looking more critically at potential correlations. However, what we do know are the number of children for whom child protection issues are a sad fact in their lives.

The current Department of Health (1991) guidance, *Working Together,* defines four types of abuse: neglect (i.e. neglect of a child or failure to thrive), physical abuse, sexual abuse, or emotional abuse. In England, there were 32 351 children on Child Protection Registers as of 31 March 1996. The bulk of these are between the ages of 1 and 9 years, and there is about an equal proportion of boys and girls. Partly as a result of the Children Act 1989, the majority of these live at home (96 per cent) with some evidence of a decline in care orders since the introduction of the new legislation. In broad terms, and in order to fix the size of the problem, there are 29 children per 10 000 of the population aged under 18 years on child protection registers. Against the background of these statistics, I now want to describe one inner-city project which, in partnership with statutory agencies, seeks to bring together mental health and child protection issues.

The Meeting Place is a small homely venue with plenty of room and an environment which seeks to put families completely at their ease. It has the appearance of a welcoming home with plenty of toys and decorations which reflect the rich cultural mix of users. While there is a growing national network of unsupervised contact, there are few centres such as The Meeting Place, which provides support and safety for families where access might be difficult or indeed dangerous. Funded by a combination of Thomas Coram's voluntary income, grants from the Inner London and Middlesex Probation Services and local authority contracts, the emphasis of the centre is always upon the child's physical safety and emotional needs.

Counselling is given to improve the quality of contact sessions for the child and, where appropriate, the aim is to move to a less supervised environment, where carers manage their own contact arrangements. Established in 1987, the project does two-thirds of its work with children who are in the care of the local authority and have been removed from their parents because of either physical, sexual, emotional abuse or neglect or because of long-term serious illness of one or both parents. The remainder of the work is made up of private law referrals, where parents have been involved in protracted and intense disputes through the court system and are unable to reach any agreement over contact arrangements. Again, suspected or actual abuse of the children is often an issue.

Both child protection and the management of mental illness are vital components of The Meeting Place's daily work. Practice involves:

1. Developing observation skills relating to children's play.
2. Building up skills to communicate with children.
3. Working in a way that facilitates contact and communication between the child(ren) and parent(s).
4. Using a range of techniques to work alongside parents with mental health difficulties in the rebuilding of a relationship.

All of this is best demonstrated by an example of The Meeting Place's work.

Case example

David is 10 years old and lives with his mother, after an acrimonious separation. Social services had been involved before the separation. Although concern had been expressed, his name had not been placed on the local child protection register. David's father was unemployed, forced to give up irregular employment in the building trade as the result of mental illness, questioningly diagnosed as schizophrenia. Unsupervised contact visits between David and his father proved impossible after an attempt at abduction and, since David still wished to maintain contact, The Meeting Place was approached. Initially, there were separate meetings with David's mother and father. These were dominated by both partners' wish to talk about the unsatisfactory nature of their relationship and the anger that remained. Gradually, it became possible to gain some acceptance that contact was first and foremost for David's benefit and that these meetings were not to be a battleground for scores to be settled.

The details of the contact were explained, with separate rooms for both parents, studious arrangements to ensure the carers did not meet and David's favourite toys placed in the room where he would have contact with his father. On the first – and indeed subsequent meetings – David began by making a glass of orange juice for himself and leaving it in the room where his mother was waiting. This provided him with an excuse to visit, both to check that his mother was all right and to reassure her that he was coping. As is frequently the case, David also tried to act as a bridge in the vain hope of bringing his estranged parents together.

During several months of contact visits, punctuated by several meetings with both parents, it became possible to demonstrate that however difficult it was for the parents, David felt reassured by contact with his father. He settled both at home and school, was relieved to see that his father was coping alone and talked to staff of his fears that he had driven the marriage apart. Eventually, it became possible to move these contact services to an unsupervised centre where both parents met for David's benefit.

Such a relatively rosy outcome is not always the case and it will be appreciated that measures of success are, at best, slippery. Over an 18-month period, from September 1994, a sample of 42 families using The Meeting Place, following court orders specifically directing supervision of contact, were followed. From the data collected it was known that in a quarter of the cases there was known child abuse of one or more children. In 6 per cent of cases children had been abducted. There had been domestic violence or severe parental conflict in 22 per cent of the families. Sixteen per cent had also involved the introduction of an unknown or long-absent parent and 10 per cent were experiencing drug and/or alcohol addiction. In 11 per cent there had been chronic mental illness diagnosed and the case notes indicated suspected mental illness in a number of other families. Of these, the courts responsible for the orders were as shown in Table 13.1.

Table 13.1 Allocation of orders by courts

County Court	40%
High Court	25%
Magistrates Court	10%
Principal Registry/Inner London Family Proceedings Court	20%

Court Welfare Officers were usually involved in the referrals to the project of the 42 families worked with during this period. What is, of course, of most significance is the outcome of The Meeting Place visits to these families (see Table 13.2).

Table 13.2 Outcomes of supervised contact at The Meeting Place

Consent order for unsupervised contact: proceedings withdrawn	36%
Unsupervised arrangements made by families: proceedings withdrawn	18%
Contact terminated by parental agreement	18%
Long term supervision	14%
Contact failed	14%
	100%

These figures demand some careful explanation. In 36 per cent of cases, contact arrangements were resolved by means of a consent order and 18 per cent of the families were eventually able to make their own arrangements, without any court orders. In addition, a further 18 per cent of parents voluntarily withdrew from court proceedings, having decided that to pursue their application for contact was not in the child's best interests. This brings us to some important principles of the work.

First, failure of contact may, in certain circumstances, be a satisfactory outcome. For many families referral to The Meeting Place is the culmination of a series of other far less satisfactory contact arrangements. A resolution of the intractable nature of the contact or a greater awareness that contact may sometimes be harmful to a child, may assist in helping the court reach a permanent decision. Clearly, in those circumstances where it has been possible to progress to unsupervised contact, then the 'success' is more tangible.

Finally, in this context, what the service – and these statistics – help to demonstrate is that a resolution of the families' problems removed from the adversarial setting of court has to be better for families. It is also more cost-effective.

Among the sampled 42 families was a referral from a County Court, concerning a family of two children, both under the age of 12 years. The mother alleged that her husband, who had custody of the two children, had a mental illness, was gay, a drug user and had sexually abused one of the children. She had consistently opposed any plans for the children and destroyed previous attempts at contact. The Meeting Place conducted, in this case, a series of pre-meetings with both parties, agreeing to offer supervised contact for the children and their mother. While the father subsequently attended with the children, the mother refused to come and subsequently withdrew her opposition to the placement.

In another situation, a father had alleged that his daughter had been sexually abused by the son of his ex-wife's new partner, who was also the father's brother-in-law. The mother steadfastly believed these allegations to be malicious and, indeed, an NSPCC investigation had revealed no evidence of abuse. The father had received a brief period of psychiatric treatment about 5 years ago but was now maintaining steady employment. The family had been badly divided by the separation; the eldest male child was with his father and the two younger siblings lived with their mother. There was little contact between the children and none at all between the children and their separated parents. Contact, through The Meeting Place, was to enable the parents to address the issues.

As a result of intervention, contact went well and continued outside a formal meeting. The eldest child was able to visit his mother and sisters at home and there was a gradual easing of the supervision for contact between the father and his daughters. When the court order for contact eventually expired, it then became possible to move to an unsupervised arrangement.

Far from representing a 'conflict of interest', The Meeting Place operates by collaboration at a number of levels: through genuine inter-agency working, involving a voluntary organization, the courts, the probation service, and local authorities.

The privilege of any voluntary organization lies in its freedom from those statutory powers which are the burden of other agencies. The responsibility that goes with that freedom is, I believe, a willingness to work alongside courts, local authorities and probation departments. Secondly, The Meeting Place represents a collaboration between carers who, over a period of time, either learn to put their differences aside in the best interests of the children or learn to accept that such collaboration is impossible.

With one in three marriages ending in divorce in the UK and approximately 100 000 children every year losing contact with one of their parents, as a result of the breakdown of the parental relationship, the project aims to provide a preventative service. Children often experience emotional damage as a result of a breakdown in the parental relationship and this can sometimes be replicated in the pattern of their relationships when they in turn become parents. Hence, any attempt to break this pattern seeks also to establish a fresh start for the future.

The Meeting Place addresses the interface of mental health and child protection in a significant percentage of seen families. To some extent, located in a voluntary childcare agency the project is, as already acknowledged, free from the statutory responsibilities of other agencies. What then are the wider issues which arise from this interface of mental health and child protection?

Of overwhelming importance must be ensuring when dealing with child protection that mental health issues are also addressed. There are some very real logistical problems which often prevent this taking place. Reference was made earlier to the lack of adequate statistical data. The increasing split in local authorities between adult and children's services does not always assist coordination. This may be further hampered by the lack of an holistic approach to childcare itself. Not only are there still significant gaps between say, health, education and social services in the provision of seamless childcare, but the growing development of contracted out services could fragment things even further. As we move closer to an American view of welfare where children's needs are broken down into stand-alone contracted services, it will be less easy to ensure that, for example, the interface of child protection and mental health problems in a family are comprehensively addressed.

In this respect, the development of children's service plans, mirroring the more established community care plans for adults, could provide an opportunity to ensure that children do not fall through welfare nets.

Of equal complexity are the fine distinctions which have to be made as to when adult mental health problems, experienced by one or both parents, become child protection issues. This is largely uncharted water and impinges in one respect on the successful campaign launched in 1995 by *Community Care* magazine on the difficulties of children who become carers.

Adult mental health problems inevitably affect the lives of children, whether as a result of new responsibilities they are expected to shoulder or, more dramatically, when adult behaviour leads to child abuse.

Lastly, we know little of those ethnically sensitive issues concerning both mental health and child protection. While there is a growing body of information informing transcultural psychiatry, there has been little work done on the interface of mental health and child protection within differing minority ethnic groups. Sensitivity to these issues needs to be reflected in much more research (see Chapter 9).

The optimism which accompanied the launch of the National Health Service is no longer with us. We have given up the belief that need is finite and can be quenched when the resources are available. Increasingly, sophisticated welfare systems detect new and often growing needs. The interface between mental health and child protection represents one of those growing needs. What remains just as important is the imperative for voluntary and statutory services to work together. The Meeting Place represents one small example of this kind of cooperation but, like the welfare state itself, it inevitably raises more new questions than it is able to answer.

14

Providing services to children and families where the parent has a mental health problem: the Australian experience

Vicki Cowling

Summary

In the past, high risk studies of children of parents with mental illness have clearly established the extent and nature of emotional and behavioural disorders in this group, but little has been done to respond with direct service provision. Parents are treated by the adult psychiatric system, which traditionally does not include a systematic response to the needs of the children of that parent, or to the needs of the patient as a *parent*. Children identified as requiring treatment become clients of the child psychiatric system, leaving many children invisible to either system. In 1993, a research project was commenced at the Early Psychosis Research Centre at The University of Melbourne, which aimed to explore and understand how parents with mental illness and their children could be effectively supported. This project was the first attempt in Australia to explore these needs and found that effective intervention for children would include support for the parent, information about the effect of mental illness on their parent and their home life, and the presence and support of an adult who could share their worries and fears. Parents require support and reassurance in their role as parent, with this provided in a flexible manner according to the fluctuation of their illness. Inter-agency collaboration is discussed as a systematic response to the issue.

'When mum got sick and we were alone with her, we didn't know where to get help. I was 9 years old. We didn't understand what was happening, and did not know who to call, except dad, but we didn't know where he was or how to ring him. We were scared of mum and what she might do . . .'

'You are unsure of who to trust. You don't know who is telling the truth. You love your mum and want to believe her, even though what she is saying sounds a bit weird, but if you don't believe your mother you feel guilty and you feel like you are deceiving her.' (A young woman who, from the age of 9 years, cared for her two younger sisters and her mother, who has schizophrenia)

Introduction

In April 1993 a research project titled 'Children of Parents Experiencing Major Mental Illness' was initiated at the Early Psychosis Research Centre, The University of Melbourne, with the focus on children of parents experiencing psychotic disorders. This specific focus occurred due to time and resource limitations. Also, many people who experience such disorders will require admission to hospital, and ongoing treatment.

This was the first attempt in Australia to address this question. More significantly, there was no clearly identified group on which to focus. Part of the process of the research was making the 'invisible' visible, and developing a culture in relation to children of parents with mental illness, and the role of parent in the lives of people traditionally identified simply as the patient, or client.

The questions addressed were: what did parents and professionals identify as the needs of the children? What did parents identify as their own support needs, and why did they not seek support?

Context

The issue is one which has always required attention on the grounds of basic human rights, the rights of children to grow up in the best possible environment, and the rights of parents to have the support required to provide this environment (UN *Convention on the Rights of the Child*, 1991, Article 18.2).

In previous eras, the mentally ill have been set apart and conferred with an inferior status. From this approach it has followed that the specific and intimate issues of sexuality, fertility, pregnancy and childbirth in this population have been ignored. Women who were institutionalized were transferred to another hospital until the birth of the baby, then returned to the psychiatric institution alone. Adoption arrangements were made for the child by the maternity unit, when no family member was available to provide care (Apfel and Handel, 1993).

More recently the shift from institutional to community care means that people with mental illness now have greater opportunity to participate in community life by choosing to form relationships and have children. This has seen an increase in the number of children born to people with mental illness (David and Morgall, 1990) which confronts all service sectors with the need to develop new ways of responding.

Identifying children and parents

Data concerning the incidence of adult psychiatric patients who also have dependent children is not routinely collected, leaving estimates to be made from census and epidemiological data. In Australia it can be roughly estimated that 27 000 children are affected. This is based on the number of women aged 20–45 years, the incidence and age of onset of schizophrenia and affective disorders, and data on the proportion of women with such disorders who have children (Gottesman, 1991).

This lack of data is not unique to Australia. Studies from the United States (Blanch *et al.*, 1994), the United Kingdom (Poole, 1996), and Denmark (Wang and Goldschmidt,

1994) report that no statistics are available to indicate what proportion of patients are parents.

Risks for children

Children of parents with psychotic disorders are at increased risk of developing such a disorder on genetic grounds (Ritsner *et al.*, 1991) and are also at increased risk of developing emotional and behavioural problems on the basis of deleterious developmental experiences (Goodman, 1984). This is more of an issue than in the past when it was more routine to take children into care, thus removing them from the negative effects associated with their parent's illness.

The emotional/behavioural problems for children do not stem in the main from the parent's mental illness, but rather from associated psychosocial disturbance in the family (Rutter and Quinton, 1984). The risks of psychological, social and educational problems arise from poverty, family discord and disorganization, including housing problems, and disruption in schooling and care due to repeated admissions of the parent to hospital (Silverman, 1989).

Some children are resilient to poor outcomes. Factors contributing to resilience include the child's temperament, the availability of one or more adults with whom the child can develop a supportive relationship, the child's age at the time of parental breakdown, a stable, cohesive family, and the extent and quality of the external support system (Garmezy *et al.*, 1984; Feldman *et al.*, 1987).

Different effects on children will be apparent at different stages of their lives. Babies may be less responsive and spontaneous, and they may be more withdrawn and apathetic. Primary school children may have low self-esteem, and also may be anxious and withdrawn. Adolescents, in becoming increasingly aware of how different home and family life is, may experience low self-confidence, isolation, and feelings of responsibility (Goldstein, 1987).

The research project

The aim of the research project was to identify the needs of both children and their parents. Inclusion criteria for each data-gathering step were: that parents had a diagnosed psychotic disorder, that they had one or more children under 18 years old, and that they had full-time custody of their children, or had regular contact.

Parents made a direct and valuable contribution to the research. In 1994 and 1995 a total of 70 parents responded to a mailout questionnaire or participated in eight focus groups. Both procedures addressed the issue of service and support needs identified by parents for themselves and their children. As parents with a psychiatric illness and their children may be clients of one or more government or non-government health and welfare agency, a mailing list of 427 of these agencies operating in Victoria was prepared. Each agency received several copies of the questionnaire and an explanatory letter requesting they distribute the questionnaire to parents. Parents were informed about the research project by a staff member and could take away the questionnaire with an accompanying Plain Language Statement and Informed Consent Statement, for completion.

The focus groups were arranged with the cooperation of service providers, who were interested in contributing to the research. Practitioners in eight community mental health or psychosocial rehabilitation settings approached parents whom they believed could contribute, and arranged the interview room for the agreed date. Numbers in the focus groups ranged from two to four parents.

The following tables (Tables 14.1 and 14.2) summarize the survey and focus group responses of parents concerning their own support needs and those of their children.

Table 14.1 Children's needs identified by their parents

Continuity of care and least disruption to home and school when parents are hospitalized

Explanation of events surrounding their parent's illness

Someone available for the child to learn to trust and talk to about fears, guilt and confusion

Programmes where children can meet with other children

Table 14.2 Parents' needs identified by parents

Continuity of relationship with supportive worker
Reassurance about quality of their parenting
Quality care for their children
Suitable place for children to visit parents in hospital
Parent support groups
Understanding of mental illness in the community, including their own families

Parents were also asked about the factors which discourage them from seeking help and support. Parents' greatest fear is that by asking for help, they will be seen as not coping and their children will be removed by child protection authorities. Also, asking for help seems like failure, when it is important to feel independent and in control.

A brief survey of service providers was also conducted. The survey was mailed to over 600 health, welfare, government and non-government agencies in the State of Victoria. A total of 136 individual responses were received.

Service providers were asked first to identify both the areas of greatest difficulty for children, and the most effective interventions. They were able to make multiple choice responses to these questions. Eighty per cent of service providers considered that 'parenting' their parent was a difficulty for children. This may include reassuring their parent, defusing emotions, managing household chores and providing physical care. Seventy-six per cent of respondents also believed that a child's lack of knowledge and understanding about their parent's mental illness is a difficulty. Other identified areas of difficulty were the concern children have about future mental illness themselves, and isolation from other children.

A final, open-ended question asked service providers to identify their own needs in relation to professional development and skills training. Service providers nominated the need for information and increased understanding about mental illness, particularly in relation to the implications for child protection. They would like to know how to talk sensitively with children about their parent's mental illness, as they are concerned that they could unnecessarily alarm or upset a child. Also nominated was training so they can work effectively with parents who do not identify or respond to their child's development needs. Resources which could help professionals work with these families included workbooks and videos.

Also conducted in 1995 were interviews with 13 parents. Some parents had participated in the earlier survey or focus groups. Others rang to ask if they could participate. The purpose of the interviews was to document the degree, and type of disruption occurring for families due to a parent's mental illness, in order to understand how that may affect children. Eleven mothers and two fathers were interviewed, with a total of 16 children. Eleven of the children were aged between 3 and 10 years; 10 were boys and most children lived with the interview parent.

Nine families involving 11 of the 16 children had experienced either the disruption associated with relationship breakdown or the involvement of child protection authorities. The degree of disruption was such that only two children in two families lived with both birth parents. For three families conflict associated with marriage breakdown and Family Court intervention resulted in loss of custody and limits on access visits between parent and child. In these three families the parent with mental illness had experienced the first episode of psychosis and hospital admission when their families were well established.

Seven parents had experienced their first episode of psychosis before becoming a parent, and had experienced far more hospital admissions than the remaining parents. One parent had been admitted 'countless' times, and another parent more than 20 times. For both parents the severity of their illness and lack of family support meant their respective children were placed in long-term alternative or substitute care as very young children. In one case the parent will have regular though infrequent access visits with her child. In the other case, parent and child were slowly reunited after the child had been in care for 10 years, during which time the parent maintained consistent contact with her child, despite having to travel long distances on many occasions.

During the interview parents were asked if they were willing to complete a behaviour checklist for their child – the Parent Rating Scale of the Behavioural Assessment System for Children (Reynolds and Kamphaus, 1992). Nine parents provided information about a total of 10 children – eight boys and two girls aged between 6 and 11 years.

Analysis of parents' responses showed that five of the children did have two or more scores which could point to possible problem areas. The most noticeable areas were hyperactivity, aggression and withdrawal. From what is understood from previous research, it could be expected that some children may have behaviour or emotional difficulties. On the other hand, parent scores for three of the 10 children were high on one or two of the adaptive or social scales, indicating their capacity to adapt to change, and competence in social skills.

While no firm conclusions can be drawn from the assessments of these 10 children, either individually, or as a group, it can be noted that where parent scores for children were satisfactory, those children had experienced least disturbance in family life. They were children of both two-parent and one-parent families, with a clearly distinguishing feature being the active involvement, in each case, of extended family.

The experience of one parent and her child illustrates the dilemma for a parent who needed help but was fearful of the possible consequences, and feared for her child who 'learnt fast'. The needs identified for parents and children reflect those described above.

This parent recognized that she was not well, as she had grown up with her own mother who has schizophrenia. While recognizing her own vulnerability, the parent did not want to seek help with her child as she was afraid he would be removed from her care. However, she subsequently acknowledged the need to ask for help and her child, aged 5 years, was placed in foster care where he remained for most of the next 9 months. From her experience, the parent believes that education and appropriate planning around a parent's mental illness would allow parents to arrange foster care placements for their children without feeling threatened that they will lose custody by doing so. In relation to children, the parent believes they need to know their parent's illness is not the child's fault. Children also need to know that the parent's mental illness affects behaviour and reactions.

When this parent herself was a child, no one explained what the problems were for her own mother, and while wanting to comfort her mother at times, she was wary of being verbally abused. Further, children should not have to look after themselves. At the age of 6 years her son was taking care of her, and managing the daily routines himself, such as getting breakfast, and preparing for school including making his lunch. In the evenings he would encourage his mother to lie down while he prepared his dinner. The parent believes that children can feel totally responsible, and afraid that their parent will get sick again, they try to do everything they can to prevent that.

When the parent was discharged from hospital, and her son returned home, a safety network was established for him, comprising a list of names and telephone numbers of family and friends whom he could ring if he was worried. This contrasts with the experience of the young person quoted at the beginning of this chapter who, as a child, with her siblings, felt very isolated and afraid, with no idea of where, and from whom, to seek support and protection.

Discussion

The information gathered from the surveys, focus groups and interviews does not provide neat answers about what should be done in practice to thoughtfully respond to the families, although there is clear recognition that the needs of children and parents are not being met. While common issues and themes can be identified, each family is unique and does not fit a cosy formula for service delivery.

For some parents and their children, the effect of serious illness such as a psychotic disorder is isolation, loss of status and marginalization. In families where this has not occurred it is encouraging to see that the extended family support available to them provides a buffer zone to protect the children and share some of the parenting role with parents. Some families are unable to utilize this family support for various reasons such as problematic relationships, or their extended family may simply be unable to help.

Through each of the research stages, parents have highlighted that they are individuals with needs specific to each family and to each stage of parenting. We need to recognize that they are parents of children who depend on them, and for whom they want the best opportunities for growing up, that they are people who also have an illness which may fluctuate, or may be chronic.

However, the problems posed in attempting to effectively support the parents and their children are too complex and the solutions too comprehensive for any one agency or organization to address alone. Inter-agency partnership and collaboration with parents and between services is one effective way to ensure that all children and parents can feel that they are fully members of their community.

Future directions

In thinking about a blueprint for identifying and responding to the needs of children and their parents there are three possible key points.

First and most immediate and obvious, is provision of programmes and services for children and parents, such as peer support programmes, counsellors skilled in helping children express their feelings about their parents' illness, and parent support programmes for parents.

Second, is the provision of education and resources for professionals so that they feel more confident in working with parents with mental illness, feel secure in speaking with children about this issue, and understand the possible impact on children of a parent's illness.

Third, is facilitating the development of inter-agency cooperation and collaboration, to ensure the needs of vulnerable children are identified and receive a response that is both planned and reactive to the fluctuations of the parent's mental illness. The needs of the families relate to a number of sectors: adult psychiatry, child psychiatry, family welfare, education, child protection to name the most immediate. Others would be services which support non-English speaking families, maternal and child health nurses and community police.

If the 'blueprint' is conceptualized as a hierarchy of need, we should first take care of the system, so the system can take care of the parents, and the parents can take care of their children (see Figure 14.1).

Figure 14.1 Families with dependent children where parents have a mental illness – response domains

Structural change – inter-agency cooperation and collaboration ↓ Education and resources for service providers ↓ Services and programmes for: parents children family members

Local developments

The Australian state of Victoria has seen shifts in these three domains in the past 2 years.

Inter-agency collaboration

Two projects addressing the need for an inter-sectoral approach have been implemented, and highlight the challenging process of culture change that is required for such an approach.[1,2] The aim of both projects was to bring together the range of services with whom parents with mental illness and their children may be involved, as outlined above. The longer term goal was that inter-agency guidelines and protocols would be developed that would facilitate a partnership approach in working with the families. The early work of similar replicated projects requires that stakeholders understand and respect the role each plays in working with the families and have shared aims and goals towards achieving inter-agency collaboration.

Education and resources for service providers

The Mental Health Branch of the Victorian Department of Human Services funded the development of a resource kit for service providers in adult mental health. The two short videos and workbook alert service providers to the parenting needs of adult mental health clients, and to the needs of their children.[3]

In Victoria, child protection is a service of the State Government. The Training Unit of the Department of Human Services periodically provides a 2-day professional development programme for workers in the child protection field.[4]

Professional development for the non-government child and family welfare sector is provided, periodically, by the author and colleagues, as private providers.

Services for parents, children and other family members

In recognition of the support parents can provide to one another in an environment of acceptance and understanding, there are now at least eight parent support groups in different localities of Melbourne. The first of these groups in fact began approximately 7 years ago and was a collaborative venture between a family welfare agency and a psychosocial rehabilitation programme.[5] A more recent parent support programme further illustrates the collaborative approach, with adult mental health, local council, family support, neighbourhood house, family welfare and charitable organizations all contributing to the development and running of this group.[6]

The parent support groups routinely gather weekly in a local community setting. Childcare is provided while parents meet to exchange news about concerns and achievements for themselves and their children, sometimes having invited speakers and participating in outings.

At present in Victoria there is one programme for parents, provided by a psychosocial rehabilitation service for families living in the south-east sector of Melbourne. The programme is funded to provide intensive, home-based, outreach support for up to 16 families at any one time. Parents have 24-hour access to support if required. Parents may attend a weekly support group which is also open to those who are not current clients of the programme.[7]

A peer support programme for children has been piloted here, and was considered of great benefit for the 17 participants, aged between 8 and 12 years.[8] The provision of ongoing peer support groups is dependent on the availability of funds, and consideration of the most viable structure and format for such groups. Work continues on developing this aspect of service provision.

The role, and needs of, spouses, partners, grandparents and other family members still awaits adequate recognition, understanding and response.

Conclusion

The cultural shift required is now under way, with clear recognition that the parenting needs of people with mental illness, and the needs of their dependent children, require a systematic response. Parents, adult offspring and children are actively contributing to this process by courageously speaking to the media, and also describing their experiences to tertiary students in social work, psychiatry and other disciplines. In doing so they are both coming to terms with their own experiences and challenging community attitudes towards people with mental illness and their families.

Notes

1. The 'Working Together' project was conducted over a 6-month period in the north-west sub-region of Melbourne, and was developed collaboratively by Broadmeadows Craigieburn Community Health Centre and the CHAMP Project Mental Health Research Institute. The project established one local inter-agency network which continues to develop.

    (CHAMP – Children and Mentally Ill Parents – was a 3-year project funded under the Commonwealth of Australia National Mental Health Project funding to pilot projects concerning children. See footnotes 3 and 8. The project was sponsored by the Mental Health Research Institute, Locked Bag 11, Parkville, Victoria, 3052.)

2. The 'Southern Partnership Project', an initiative of the author, was conducted over a 12-month period and aimed to develop four inter-agency networks in the southern region of Melbourne. (The Project was funded by the Victorian Health Promotion Foundation and sponsored by the School of Social Work, the University of Melbourne, Parkville, Victoria, 3052.)

3. Resource kit: *Hidden Children* video targeted to adult mental health workers; *Hard Words* video targeted to parents, children and other family members and carers, and Manual. Sponsored jointly by the CHAMP Project/Mental Health Research Institute and Department of Human Services.

4. 'Working with Parents who have a Mental Illness' focuses on risk factors associated with psychiatric illness, key issues in protective interventions and case management challenges, and includes a presentation by a parent who has mental illness.

5. The Boomerang Club, Moonee Ponds and Abercare Family Support Services, Niddrie, Victoria, 3124.
6. 'Parenting Together' is sponsored by Anglicare Family Centre and supported by Peninsula Health Care Network Psychiatric Services, Orwil Street Community House, the Brotherhood of St. Lawrence, and Frankston Council, Victoria 3199.
7. Mothers Support Programme, Prahran Mission, Prahran, Victoria, 3168.
8. Peer Support Programme, CHAMP Project, Mental Health Research Institute.

Acknowledgements

Much of the material in this chapter was first published in *Family Matters,* **45** (1996), the journal of the Australian Institute of Family Studies.

The research project described was completed while the author was a Senior Research Assistant at the Early Psychosis Research Centre, the University of Melbourne. Professor David A. Hay, Department of Psychology, Curtin University, Western Australia, was Chief Investigator. The project was funded by the Victorian Health Promotion Foundation.

Managing strategies for change in childcare and mental health services in Bath and North East Somerset

Maurice Lindsay, Robert G. Potter and Annie Shepperd

Introduction

This chapter is based upon a presentation to the UK-based Michael Sieff Foundation Conference 'Keeping Children in Mind' in September 1997 with the title 'Managing Strategies for Change'. The theme of the conference was to consider how agencies working with families must ensure that neither the needs of an adult (with mental health difficulties) nor the needs of a child are lost sight of when different perspectives are adopted and conflicts of interest can arise. The presentation focused upon the experience of adult mental health and childcare workers in both our agencies (Health and Social Services) in Bath and North East Somerset.

Bath and North East Somerset is a new unitary authority to the south of Bristol. The Authority was created as a result of local government reorganization in 1995 when the proposal to merge Wansdyke District Council, Bath City Council and the County Services from Avon County Council was agreed.

The new unitary authority began life in April 1996 having brought together three organizations with different cultures, different values, different ways of organizing services, and certainly very different aspirations.

It was the experience gained from the first case example detailed below that prompted us to look closely at the practice within our own agencies. It was also evident that we needed to examine how we worked across agencies. The fact that Bath and North East Somerset was a very new unitary authority with a newly created directorate of Housing and Social Services (and new management teams at Director, second and third tiers), and that consequently new working relationships were being established with the Health Trusts and Health Authority, gave impetus to this process. Both agencies were committed to looking at how we provided services and worked in partnership. The proposed presentation to the Sieff Conference added further fuel. The fact that the authors quickly established a working relationship and a commitment to change meant that the momentum could be maintained.

Lessons from experience

Case 1

Both the adult mental health services and childcare services from the Directorate of Housing and Social Services had been working with this particular family for a number of years. The mother was a lone parent with a long history of depression. The Directorate provided support to maintain the parent within the community and the children within the family home. On a number of occasions respite foster care was provided for the children to give the mother planned breaks and also when she was admitted to hospital for treatment. Community-based support was provided to enable the family to re-unite after such episodes. Community and hospital-based mental health staff had also been involved in providing services for the parent.

During the course of 1996 circumstances deteriorated markedly. The parent's mental health problems became more acute: she spent longer periods in hospital, including compulsory admissions. The childcare agencies became increasingly concerned about her ability to parent her children safely and meet their developing needs. Care proceedings were initiated. After consultation with the hospital-based health staff, the childcare social worker advised the parent of these proceedings and the proposed plans for the future care of the children. This was done in conjunction with the hospital-based staff, including the consultant psychiatrist. No formal planning meeting was held for the children because of concerns about the parent's fragile mental health. An application for Interim Care Orders was made to the local Family Court.

In parallel with this, the parent appealed against the decision to make her the subject of a Section 3 Order under the Mental Health Act. The Mental Health Review Tribunal requested a report from the Directorate of Housing and Social Services and this was compiled by an adult mental health social worker. When compiling her report, this social worker was apparently not given any reason to believe that the childcare arrangements would be any different from previous occasions. The parent did not say anything about care proceedings; nor did the hospital staff. The childcare case was in the process of being transferred to a new social worker. The hospital staff were firmly of the opinion that the parent's mental health difficulties were exacerbated by not being with her children. Indeed, the children were seen as a therapeutic tool to help the mother feel better and to improve her mental health.

The childcare social worker asked if she ought to attend the tribunal, but was advised by the consultant psychiatrist that this was not necessary, as in his opinion, the childcare issues were separate to the parent's mental health situation. Consequently, when the tribunal took place:

- The parent stated that the fact that her children had been taken away affected her mental health, and if this was not the case, she would be better and could return home.
- The mental health social worker said that she could not comment about this or the childcare plans.
- The consultant psychiatrist made no reference to the discussion that the childcare social worker and he had had with the parent regarding care proceedings.

Not unexpectedly the tribunal felt that it did not have sufficient information to make a decision, adjourned its hearing and requested the attendance of a senior manager at the next hearing to 'explain the rationale of the management of this case and to say what proposals there are for the future'. This is indeed what happened and the director was subpoenaed to London.

It was very evident from this case that there had been a significant breakdown in communication between and within agencies and that each service had focused on the needs of *their* client. There were different perceptions of need. One service saw the adult, the other saw the children. On the one hand professionals such as the community support worker, the community psychiatric nurse, the mental health social worker, hospital staff, the consultant psychiatrist and the general practitioner were working with the adult with mental health difficulties. On the other hand the childcare social worker, the community care worker, the family centre, the foster carers and the school were working with the children, who needed care and protection. There seemed to be an invisible barrier to communication with nobody crossing that barrier in this particular case.

This was a complex and quite extreme case and when it went wrong the effect was dramatic and certainly high profile. The case brought the problems to our attention and forced us to look at them. In doing so, we quickly became aware that this lack of communication and working together between childcare and mental health services went right through all of the respective agencies – and not just in severe or extreme cases.

In looking at the way forward, we found the Office of Public Management briefing paper 'Joint Commissioning for Child Protection' (Evans and Miller, 1995) to be particularly helpful – with its injunction to mental health practitioners to 'see the child' and to childcare practitioners to 'see the adult'. This did not appear to be happening within our agencies. We discovered what we have termed 'silo' thinking, in which childcare staff see only the child, adult care staff see only the adult, and never the twain shall meet. In considering how we got to this position we firmly pointed the finger at the effects of specialization both within and across agencies. The specialization in children's services and adult mental health services, while it had created many opportunities for service development had, at the same time, introduced barriers that families and individuals living in our communities cannot make sense of. It is clear to us that these barriers really exist, as well as being perpetuated by people who work in our organizations. Associated with this has been:

- The mystique that has developed around the services.
- The fear of making mistakes.
- Perceived deskilling – staff believing that they do not have the basic skills to assess the adult as well as the child, and vice versa.
- Avoiding such assessments and decisions because of the apparent deskilling ('it's your job to make decisions about risks to children; my job to make decisions about risks to adults').
- The establishment of blinkered services that focus upon their own clients.
- Segmented services that have found it difficult to work together.

The irony is, of course, that there are so many parallels between the services – both are high profile, both are involved in significant risk management, both have experience of the blame culture. At this stage we appeared to be facing an uphill struggle, with a high profile (but not exclusive) example of how we got things wrong. We needed to respond to this position and in doing so build upon the positives and strengths that had been equally evident in other areas of our work.

Case 2

An example where things worked better related to a lone parent mother in her late 20s with four children. A child psychiatrist had been asked by the court to prepare a report on the needs of the children. The mother had not been cooperative with the court and had not turned up on more than one occasion. At times the children had to be accommodated because their mother felt unable to cope, and then she felt guilty and a worthless failure as a mother. Her supportive childcare social worker felt there may be more to this problem and she discussed with the child psychiatrist the relevance of the maternal grandmother's history of bipolar affective disorder. During the assessment of the mother and children, the child psychiatrist felt that she was indeed developing a bipolar mood disorder and, not surprisingly, when she was depressed she was less able to care for her children. The oldest child, of 9 years, then took on a caring role both to the mother and her siblings.

It was clear that this mother's own childhood experience had been identical to that of her oldest child, with her having to take responsibility for caring for her younger siblings. She wanted to avoid facing what was happening to her perhaps out of fear that she would become as ill as her mother. As a consequence, she avoided contact with mental health services. A care plan was worked out involving the GP, adult mental health services and child and family mental health services. The childcare social worker continued to support the mother in getting help for her own mental health problems, working across role boundaries. The consultant psychiatrist was able to help the mother make the transition into adult mental health services since she felt she could trust him, because his report to the court had addressed her needs *and* the needs of the children. The primary care team took a pivotal role in this coordination. This was a case that seemed to work well, due to people cooperating in crossing boundaries.

Case 3

Another, more complicated case, involving two boys, one at junior school and one at secondary school, was referred to child and family mental health services by the childcare social worker. Both parents had longstanding mental health problems, including postnatal depression in the mother, and were in contact with adult services. One of the boys had significant emotional problems and was resident in a special school. The other was looked after by foster carers. The child and family mental health services began to address the issues of the whole family, particularly what it had been like for these children to have a mother with mental health problems, a suggestion which had come from the parents. In the first session, which was difficult for them, the mother came from the inpatient unit for the work to be done with the family. This was possible because the nurse on that unit, the mother's own keyworker, was able to prepare her for coming across and to help her deal with the issues afterwards. The joint work between child and adult mental health services and the social services and the residential school continued following the mother's discharge from hospital, with positive progress for the family. Plans are well established for one boy to return home from foster care.

The way forward

Drawing upon our experience from the cases highlighted, we recognized the importance of introducing change to the way in which our services operated, if we were going to avoid the mistakes previously made and, more importantly, build upon the positives and the good practice that had been equally evident in these cases. So we entered the change arena and resolved to avoid the impasse encapsulated in the quote 'Change is cool, you go first'. We asked ourselves some simple questions:

- Do people see the need for change?
- Whether they do or not, do they want to change?
- Do we have the climate in which to effect change?
- Do we have the impetus for change?

From our experience and discussions at a senior management level, we believed this to be the case and sought a wider perspective by undertaking a straightforward survey of frontline staff and managers that focused upon their experience of how childcare and adult mental health services had worked together to provide services to the *same* family. This research confirmed that key elements in the change equation were present, i.e. that people were dissatisfied with how things currently operated, that we had a clear vision of how things could be and that we had some practical ideas for the first steps to take. Change was needed and wanted, the climate was right, and the impetus was there. We felt that we could move forward. We recognized that both system change and culture change needed to take place.

The theme underpinning our strategies for change has been 'see the adult' *and* 'see the child'. This must be the focus at every level within each organization and between organizations. In our opinion there are a number of key issues that must be addressed to effectively manage strategies for change and realize solutions:

1. What is the quality of our collaborative working? Inter-agency – between social services, community and hospital-based mental health services. Intra-agency – between the childcare teams and adult mental health teams in social services; between the community-based and hospital-based mental health services.
2. Is there commitment at the top of our organization and does this run through our organization? Is there a similar commitment across and between our agencies? Who has an overview at senior management level? Within the Directorate of Housing

and Social Services, the Head of Assessment and Commissioning Services (Assistant Director level) has responsibility for both childcare and adult care services. The Group Managers are specialists. Within the Health Trust, both the current Chief Executive and the Operations Director have social work backgrounds in child protection and childcare. As an organization the Trust knows what 'the other side' is doing and why.

3. Does our organizational structure hinder or help us to achieve greater integration? We must consider whether we have structural flaws that we have to overcome. Does the simple location of staff or the layout of offices help or hinder us? Does our structure make it possible for strategies to be put into practice at the grass roots operational level or not?

4. How do we empower our staff (and service users)? Equally important, how do we ensure that we do not disempower them. We must consider how we will involve our staff in this change of culture and how we enable grass root practitioners to get together.

5. How do our services integrate (given that they are very distinct specialisms)? Do our childcare and adult mental health teams talk to each other? Do they work together? What are our strategies for getting health and social services to work together to provide and develop services.

6. Do our children's services plans and community care plans exist as separate entities or do they come together and plan integrated services? We need to ask the simple question – does our children's services plan include provision for services to parents with mental health problems? At the time of our presentation to the Sieff Conference, our own children's services plan did not.

It is one thing to identify the key issues but a quite different task to start taking effective action. The immediate questions that occur are – where do we start? and how do we pull others into this? We would respond by saying that you must focus on what you do in your own agency *but* you must talk to each other and work together. Our first steps included the simple task of actually debating the issues at senior management level within each of our agencies *and* between agencies *and* being determined to achieve solutions. The following actions were taken:

1. We started the wider debate by undertaking a survey of frontline staff's experiences of how childcare and adult mental health services worked together to provide services to the same family and sought ideas about what worked well and why. We sought ideas about how things could be further improved. We wanted those individual examples of good collaborative working to become the norm.

2. We established a multi-agency childcare/mental health forum with the task of drafting policies and procedures to coordinate childcare and adult mental health services. The forum has comprised community-based childcare and health and mental health staff, education welfare officers, consultant psychiatrists and hospital-based staff and service users.

3. In January 1997, the local authority established a multi-agency working party to plan the refocusing of children's services. A conference held in July 1997 launched

the refocusing debate. Workshops were held to consider the interface between childcare and adult mental health services. The conference was attended by staff at all levels from all agencies and by members of the Social Services, Housing and Education Committees of the Local Authority and representatives of the Health Authority. The debate was under way and has been widespread. It has been continued in a series of childcare and mental health seminars.

4. Within the Directorate of Housing and Social Services we have made arrangements for adult mental health service social workers to work with the childcare duty officers in the Referral and Assessment Team. Each social worker will get this experience; close links are being established and joint visits and assessments undertaken. Similarly, childcare social workers will be working with the mental health duty team and the approved social worker service. This experience will be included in induction programmes for all new members of staff and built into performance appraisal and personal development plans for all staff. The use of secondments is also encouraged. We have also established identified consultants within each childcare and mental health team for members of each service to draw upon. We have set up systems to encourage joint pieces of work – for the assessment of the need for services and the delivery of those services. Mental health staff are included in the core group of workers for child protection cases; childcare staff are involved in care planning/discharge meetings for parents.

5. The Mental Health Trust contributes to a good GP training scheme and many of the GPs specifically request to be given child and family mental health experience. Many doctors who have trained locally go on to practise locally. The local child and family mental health team is now receiving at least one referral a week, from GPs and inpatient units, relating to a family with an adult mental health problem with the question 'what can you do to help us in working with them?' Clear routes for consultation and referral have been established.

6. As a newly combined Directorate, the Directorate of Housing and Social Services have integrated the provision of childcare, adult mental health and housing services to children and parents. They provide support to avoid the loss of tenancies by adults with mental health difficulties. They no longer place parents with children in bed-and-breakfast or hostel accommodation.

7. The simple fact that childcare social workers are beginning to help children keep in touch with their parents in hospital has been an amazing trigger for referrals coming from the adult service. Seeing the child means that they are much less likely to be ignored, since previously they never went near the admission wards.

8. Joint staff training is under way within the multi-agency child protection training programme and the overall training programme for the Authority. This training initiative is firmly supported by the Area Child Protection Committee.

What progress has been made?

The first case study outlined in this chapter provided the impetus for change. Our local circumstances added strength to this as did the commitment of those at a senior level within our agencies and the enthusiasm of those at grass roots level. We do, however, feel that we are still at the beginning of the process of change and that that change is likely to be evolutionary rather than a big bang. The commitment and enthusiasm is clear; the time and capacity to put this into operation is not always so obviously available. Change would be most effectively achieved if we were in a position to nominate a post that could take full responsibility for coordinating these new joint services. The most likely scenario, which we expect will be common to most other agencies, is that existing staff will have to add these new requirements to their existing range of responsibilities.

From our positions as consultant psychiatrist and group manager (children's services) we have been able to establish effective networks so that our proposals have an impact, and are implemented, at the operational level. We are also able to use existing systems to monitor the ongoing development of coordinated services – for example through the role played by the group manager in the reviewing of all child protection cases and 'looked after' children plans. We are also undertaking a further survey of frontline staff and managers to establish another view of how experiences and perceptions have changed since the first survey in June 1997. Within the refocusing of our children's services, we are developing protocols for agencies working with children in need and parents with mental health difficulties, built upon existing good practice within and between our own agencies.

The greatest challenge has been to keep the momentum going when there are so many other pressures and demands on time. Our strategy has been to bring more and more people into the process and to use prompts such as joint training, seminars and conferences and the recognition of good practice to move things forward. We would acknowledge that change has continued but not necessarily as a managed process. What is very evident is that people's thinking has changed and that with continuing prompts their actions and practices are changing and the impetus for change is well established. The most encouraging response has been that people have not said 'we do that already' but have asked 'what can we do differently?'

Conclusion

In planning a way forward we would recommend the following:

– Avoid over-focusing on your own agency.
– Avoid merely creating different silos.
– Avoid starting the debate but not doing anything about it – nothing is more demotivating.
– On the other hand do not become complacent. Do not just get change going, keep it going and plan how you will sustain it.

Finally, consider what militates against collaborative working. A useful way of doing this is to ask your staff to brainstorm 'How can we make things worse?' List the suggestions, stop doing these and thereby effect immediate improvements. Some of the ideas that we became aware of through using this process could certainly help you to thwart collaborative working and are listed for your information:

- Do everything by phone.
- Do not confirm anything in writing.
- Believe in intuition.
- Presume everybody else knows what you are doing.
- Assume everybody is doing what they should be doing.

In our local experience, what appeared to be negatives did in fact lead us along the road to solutions. By employing the strategies and implementing the practical actions outlined in this chapter, we have begun to establish greater confidence in collaborative working between childcare and mental health services and have considered how we can build upon this. 'See the adult' and 'see the child' is not merely a theme. It underpins our thinking, planning and service delivery.

Building bridges: lessons for the future

Anthony Douglas

Discussion about how best to meet the needs of parents with mental health problems and the consequences for their children is not a new issue. Research into this has gone on for most of this century (Falkov, 1997). However, a balanced view of the needs of both parents and children is much newer.

Having a mental health problem does not in itself mean that your children will be more vulnerable or even in danger. As Channi Kumar put it:

> 'Most mentally ill mothers don't abuse children and most abusive mothers are not considered mentally ill'.   (Kumar, personal communication, 1997)

However, the incapacity of some parents resulting from their mental health problems does pose serious risks and difficulties for their children. The nature of these risks range widely from homicide to insufficient care and attention, leading to impairments in health and development. It is still the case that most parents who have mental health problems are responsible and caring parents. There are many examples in this book of how well parents have coped and of the various strategies they have adopted in order to do so.

The professionals and agencies who see families in the community all have a responsibility to support children and their families. Given the enormous variation in the degree and nature of the needs which exist, it is crucial that 'working together' acts as the key operational principle between professional organizations. No one can practice safely or sensitively alone in this area because the whole picture has to be put together and because no one has – in a world of increasing specialization – all the skills and knowledge required. The other reason for promoting inter-agency collaboration is that there are significant ethical and legal issues to consider and to weigh up in any intervention in family life, as Liz Sayce has discussed earlier in Chapter 5.

Freud said that those who forget the past are condemned to repeat it. The same is true of the child protection/adult mental health interface. A selection of the most serious cases reported and reviewed in 1995, 1996 and 1997 reveal that the same mistakes highlighted in previous cases are recurring, with sufficient repetition to be indicative of a deep and continuing malaise. When a child is killed, investigators should always consider if the parent had a mental health problem, however disguised. In Chapter 5, Liz Sayce warned of the dangers of denying full citizenship to people with mental health problems, including the right to parent. We also cannot avoid the uncomfortable reality of serious child protection cases. Whilst drawing material from investigations and inquiries where a child dies can be criticized for skewing 'the big picture' negatively or pessimistically, assumptions made and decisions taken by professionals in numerous other cases will have avoided fatal consequences by chance rather than by design.

Tragic coincidence is of course a feature of complex childcare cases and indeed complex mental health cases. Many children die because of a split-second loss of control, even if the background factors make such a loss of control in their own family more likely than in the average family. A number of recent cases in which a parent has killed their children and then themselves, often following marital breakdown, have received considerable publicity. In one such tragedy, in June 1997, an accountant, John Chetwynd, jumped off Beachy Head with his sons, Kevin, aged 3 years, and Christopher, aged 9 years, after a violent assault on his Vietnamese wife. The case left more questions than answers, especially about family violence (Toolis, 1998). Other children and families with the same background features manage to avoid the same adverse factors tragically combining in a single fatal incident. We often underestimate how important professional contact can be to families, in reducing the risk of the specific forces in a specific family merging fatally. On the other hand, some parents and indeed some single adults carry out their threat, made to professionals, to kill a child. These are some of the most desperate situations professionals encounter, because the adults involved often refuse to cooperate with all professional interventions. There are seldom grounds for compulsorily detaining or prosecuting these adults in advance of them committing the inevitable serious crime.

The following examples illustrate some of these recurring themes. Chapter 1 of this book started with a quote from *The Times* in February 1997 – 'A baby on an at-risk register was thrown to his death by his mentally ill mother after social services decided she was fit to care for him. Daniel Whayman, aged 16 weeks, died after his mother Lisa, 33, threw him from the 150 feet Orwell Bridge near Ipswich'. In fact, Lisa Whayman had collected Daniel in a taxi from her own mother's house. She told the taxi driver to drop her off at the Orwell Bridge, a high and wide bridge known locally as a popular suicide location. The taxi driver, a bit-part player, asked no questions and drove straight off. The childcare social worker began by being angry with the mother for what she had done, seeing her as bad. It was only later that professionals realized just how mentally ill she was.

The second example is from a London duty desk. A childcare social worker is following up an allegation made through the local newspaper that a woman is procuring children for her live-in partner, a Schedule 1 offender. The journalist asks if there is a paedophile ring operating, another sign of the times. The childcare worker diligently follows up the allegation and quizzes the mother about her relationship. Later the same day, the mother attempts suicide. Unbeknown to the childcare social worker, the mother is on the caseload of a mental health team social worker in her own right, for depression. As with many such examples, there was no particular warning sign and the social worker was not to blame. Yet a simple check would have identified this additional dimension. In fact, there was no paedophile ring.

The third example is a sentence taken from a letter written by a housing officer to a Director of Social Services in a South of England county: 'I confirm that complaints have been received from neighbours that Mrs D is in the habit of leaving her children alone and unattended for lengthy periods during the day. This woman's mental state is a cause for concern although the two children are bright and cheerful. Please would you advise me of the outcome of your enquiries.' The outcome of this case was that there were no child protection concerns once the mother had been supported to find a childminder and once a small level of financial support had been given. In this case, an assessment of the children's situation in the round was needed, of which the child protection component turned out to be a minor part. Most parents with mental health problems bring their children up successfully, despite the occasional bad times.

Another recent case illustrates the importance of investigatory techniques within assessment processes. Darren Carr was a 25-year-old man, who developed schizophrenia in his early 20s whilst in Berkshire. He tried to kill his mother with a hammer but was only charged with a breach of the peace, although he did receive a forensic assessment and good psychiatric care for a period of time in a medium-secure unit and then in a community hostel. When he moved counties, Berkshire's services gradually lost touch with him, although they were still worried about what he might do. In Abingdon, Oxfordshire, he moved in with a woman and her two children, as a live-in nanny. There is no legal requirement for nannies to be registered under the Children Act to provide day care. A few months later, he set fire to the house, killing the woman and her two young children. Mental health services in Berkshire had referred Carr to childcare services in Oxfordshire, but staff in Oxfordshire had not followed up the concerns by making adequate checks. An assumption was made that because Carr was not a Schedule 1 offender, he was not 'dangerous'. In fact, the children had previously been on the Oxfordshire child protection register for different reasons.

Had the information available been properly collated and evaluated, or if a risk assessment had been carried out in which the relevance of certain bits of information had been weighed up, things may have turned out differently. Carr was subject to continuing diagnostic uncertainty. One of the recommendations of the external inquiry was that 'Oxfordshire Social Services Department should provide refresher training in mental health, particularly in relation to psychopathic disorder and forensic psychiatry, to all workers within the Oxfordshire Child Protection and Families Division' (*Report of the Inquiry into the Treatment and Care of Darren Carr*, 1997).

Finally, one of the saddest and perhaps the most horrific case of all. On his 32nd birthday, Shaun Anthony Armstrong sexually assaulted and killed a 3-year-old girl, Rosie Palmer, in Hartlepool. She had gone out to buy an ice-cream from a van about 40 yards from her home only to be raped and murdered by Armstrong. The van had stopped outside his house, and he bought her the ice-cream. Armstrong pleaded guilty to sexual assault and murder at Leeds Crown Court in 1995 and was sentenced to life imprisonment.

The seeds of what happened were sown early in Armstrong's life. His father was in fact his grandfather, and his mother was 18 years old when she gave birth to him as a result of this incestuous relationship. After an isolated early childhood, his mother started to sexually abuse him when he was 7 years old, and this abuse progressed to full sexual intercourse when he was 13 years old. He saw various psychologists and psychiatrists as a child. After leaving school, he joined the Navy but was discharged as unfit, and then had a series of temporary jobs. He was frequently convicted of burglaries, thefts and dishonesty offences. Aged 22 years, he tried to commit suicide. He had a number of psychiatric assessments and admissions to psychiatric units in his 20s and early 30s. The attempted suicides continued. He also had a drink and drugs problem. It was alleged he sexually abused more than one young girl before he killed Rosie Palmer. His attempts to take his own life continued in Wakefield Prison after he had been sentenced to life imprisonment.

An independent panel of inquiry found that local mental health services had not cared adequately for Armstrong during the critical years preceding Rosie Palmer's murder, but that her death could neither have been predicted nor prevented (*Report of the Panel of Inquiry Presented to the Tees District Health Authority into the Treatment and Care of Sean Armstrong*, 1996).

Rosie's mother, Beverley Palmer, queried this and unsuccessfully sued the Health Authorities responsible for Armstrong's care. She claimed there were at least 15 specific warnings that if Armstrong was released from hospital, he would kill a child. It is possible that if the criminal intelligence about Armstrong's history of sexual offences and his statements in hospital to nursing staff had been shared between the hospital, the police and social services, there might have been a greater realization of what he might do. Nothing predicts future behaviour better than past behaviour.

In a recent major study, Dr Adrian Falkov reviewed a selection of child protection inquiry reports and found that one in three child murders are committed by adults with mental health problems, mostly within the family. Whatever happened to Shaun Anthony Armstrong as a child destroyed not only his life but Rosie Palmer's and those who cared about her. Like many other child abusers, Armstrong was abused as a child and began abusing others at the same time as he was being abused himself. The two went hand in hand. He needed help as a child with unrecognized mental health problems and then as a young abuser. The only help Rosie Palmer needed was for Armstrong to be contained or cured before he met her. Her mother, Beverley Palmer, like Armstrong, attempted suicide on 10 occasions after Rosie's death, through sheer grief (*Observer*, 10 August 1997).

These cases are shocking in themselves, yet being shocked does not help us to understand how mistakes are repeatedly made by professional staff who in hindsight are as shocked as everyone else, and who blame themselves and feel a great sense of guilt irrespective of whether any disciplinary action is taken against them for their mistakes.

At one level, we should not ask the impossible. It is far from simple to map someone's state of mind. It is not always easy to understand the thoughts and intentions of close partners, let alone the game plan of individuals as complex as the parents described in these case examples. What was going through Armstrong's mind as he killed Rosie Palmer? Through Darren Carr's mind? Through Lisa Whayman's mind? This is a question all of us involved with child protection and mental health need to try to understand. It is not just a question for forensic adult psychiatrists and psychologists after the event. And as well as improving our awareness of the mind-set of people who threaten children, we need to be aware of our own mind-set which, as these case examples demonstrate, can at times be totally unaware of what is really going on.

The role of social workers in serious child protection cases is similar to that of police officers. In this area of work, their task is to prevent a serious crime being committed. But most detectives would not be where they are today without paid informants. Even with informants, the clear-up rate for offences is low. Why should society expect social workers to have a better clear-up rate than trained detectives? With the growing emphasis on evidence-based social work, use of paid informants is worth thinking about. Whilst it is morally problematic to encourage a society of snitchers, who ring in on free helplines to report everything from benefit fraud to noise nuisance, the damage done to the image of social services by not realizing what has actually been going on in serious childcare cases, means traditional methods of investigation and assessment may need to be modernized.

In Chapters 11 and 12 of this book the emphasis was placed on the need for greater awareness and training. Those needs of course remain eternally valid. The Department of Health has now commissioned a new and most welcome training pack on Child Protection and Mental Health. Training is one implication for organizations, but only one. Policy issues also need clarifying, although I remain unconvinced that the current climate of zero tolerance is illuminating new policy guidance. In July 1997, the government issued national policy guidelines for working with parents who misuse drugs. In general, there is disapproval of drug users who have, or want to have, children. Understandable, but possibly of little help to those working with parents, or to those parents and indeed their children.

One of the common factors in the cases I have described is that they were not accorded the highest priority at the defining moment. Those cases which do achieve premier league status, full of emergencies and crises, often with a sensational edge to them, are generally handled well. Each agency pulls all the stops out. However, dealing with the top-drawer cases seems to exhaust all available energy. Routine everyday cases are much more likely to be subject to boundary disputes, dumping between teams, and a reluctance by any one worker to 'catch and carry' the case any distance. The perception, or the reality, of insufficient capacity to take on any more stress and pressure may lie behind this phenomenon. Teams tend to rationalize their workload to fit it into the staff capacity they have at any one time. That can lead to decisions to exclude rigorous assessments of some cases that would be allocated in easier times. Team managers in social services departments carry out this juggling act every day. Some of them, punch-drunk from this relentless assault, find it hard to maintain their equilibrium, confidence and judgement. Organizations tend to see the development of managers in terms of leadership, team-working and creative thinking. But in child protection work and mental health work there is no substitute for having a number of senior staff looking at the workload and thinking through the risks on specific cases. This can either be senior practitioners along with the team manager, or experienced social workers, or more senior managers. All too often, the first-line manager is left alone. Even worse, if the first-line manager is not up to it, social workers can be left entirely to their own devices.

In the case examples given, the conflict of interest between the needs of children and the needs of parents stands out. Inside the same organization, mental health staff can advocate for the very parent who threatens the well-being of the same child whom childcare staff are attempting to protect. The conflict of interest, rather than being resolved, is reproduced amongst professionals. Identifying a sense of common purpose across the child protection/mental health divide needs to replace confrontational advocacy as a paradigm. That can only come from considering the needs of both child and parent as a whole, even when they are in conflict. All too often, child protection meetings turn into one-sided displays of the professional elitism of childcare staff, at which other professionals with points of view are made to feel spectators.

At the other end of the spectrum, mental health case conferences can seem like a whistle-stop tour of cases, rarely stopping to look at any one in any depth. The reviewing mechanisms for each are very different, and the professional relationships within each area are different. The relationship between psychiatrists and CPNs is crucial in mental health work, and is a rarely researched area sometimes fraught with tensions. Similarly, the relationship between childcare staff in social services and teachers, vital to monitoring school-age children, is complicated and too easily taken for granted. Partnership working comes only if each partner puts something into and gets something out of the encounter, so they have a stake in the outcome. One member of staff in a joint financed inter-agency team put it quite simply – 'All of us from our different agencies feel this is *our* service'.

To be effective, a child protection system, and a mental health system, have to make sense to each member agency, and have to help them with their own often overwhelming internal agenda. The same goes for the child protection/mental health system. If it is not in place, it has to be assembled so as to make sense to education professionals, social services professionals, and health service professionals. What is true between agencies is true within agencies, where the specialist divide can be equally intense.

As far as assessments are concerned, the implications for organizations are that a generic approach to assessment might be better than the current exclusively specialist focus, all-round vision rather than tunnel vision. A single referral may contain childcare needs, mental health needs, a carer's needs, possibly substance misuse, and even a youth crime aspect if the parent is especially young. Similarly, in other service-user groups, a single referral may contain potential information about the needs of an older person, learning disability needs, and again the needs of a carer. It is more realistic for all assessments, certainly in social services but also in nursing agencies, to contain a checklist of the major areas to cover. Professionals need to develop the skills and confidence to work across service-user group boundaries.

Children's needs are not always immediately apparent. Some children are more resilient than others and are able to survive despite considerable adversity (see Chapter 2). For example, Charlie Chaplin's mother went into a mental hospital in 1901 when he was 12 and Charlie spent the rest of his childhood fending for himself and successfully avoiding being taken into care.

Childcare assessments are better done in the round. A child protection investigation should perhaps always be part of a holistic child-in-need assessment. That approach is more likely to lend itself to the appreciation of complexity. In general terms, this would involve a shift in emphasis from investigating whether children are at risk of abuse from the parenting of their mentally ill parents towards a starting-point of considering whether the parents have problems in parenting arising from their mental ill-health. This wider focus then has to be narrowed down to a child protection focus at the point or for the period in which children's lives are in obvious danger.

We are still in a muddle about confidentiality. In the Darren Carr case, the social worker in Berkshire was not sure whether passing on information to Oxfordshire would constitute a betrayal of Carr's confidence. His team leader overruled him, but it is clear that a lot of information is not passed on because a professional decision is made, rightly or wrongly, to withhold it. The issue is not resolved at a national level. The National Health Services Executive (NHSE) continues to advise Health Trusts that it cannot share patient information with a local authority, even when joint provision between the Trust and the local authority is being established for a specific service.

The need for change should not just be laid at the door of social workers. When there is an inquiry, the rabbits in the headlights are usually the social workers. Other professions become invisible when things go wrong. In a recent inquiry in Sheffield, after a child died, one of the recommendations to doctors was that : 'Any doctor (GP) who knows that a patient with a mental health problem is caring for a child must ensure the safety of the child.' The role of GPs is rarely explored as the crucial determinant of under-recognition or misdiagnosis in a child protection case. An implication for organizations of many of the cases I have illustrated is the need for doctors to ensure medical responsibility is properly handed over, either across Health Authority boundaries or between a hospital or a specialist unit and community health services.

The lessons to learn from the cases in this concluding chapter are inter-agency lessons, but the inter-agency scene these days is characterized by formalized fragmentation, both within local agencies and across the Civil Service and government departments. The devastation caused by organizational change on professional lives is rarely featured in the dissection of mistakes. Professional staff can easily be mesmerized by what is happening in their workplaces and distracted from their primary focus. Corporate approaches and consensus-building at the local level – seeing service users in the round rather than each separate agency seeing a small and separate part – are far from easy, but they have to be developed if services are to be connected up, and children and adults are to be properly supported and protected.

If the note on which our book ends is a pessimistic one, this is not incompatible with some of the positive work and developments described throughout the text. Understanding the difficulties and complexities of child protection and mental health work is a prerequisite for putting the right type of services in place. A conflict of interest yes, but ultimately a resolvable one, as so many of our contributors have shown.

Bibliography and further reading

Abbott, P. and Sapsford, R. (1987). *Community Care of Mentally Handicapped Children*. Milton Keynes: Open University Press.

Acock, A.C and Demo, D.A (1994). *Family Diversity and Well Being*. Sage: London.

Adams, J., McCllelan, J., *et al*. (1995). 'Sexually inappropriate behaviours in seriously mentally ill children and adolescents', *Child Abuse and Neglect,* **19**(5), 555–568.

Adcock, M. (1996). 'A legal framework for child protection: The Children Act 1989 (UK)'. In: M. Gopfert, J. Webster and M.V. Seeman (Eds) *Parental Psychiatric Disorder: Distressed Parents and their Children*. Cambridge: Cambridge University Press.

Addison, C. (1988). *Planning Investigative Projects: A Workbook for Social Services Practitioners*. London: National Institute for Social Work.

Ainsworth, M.D.S., Blehar, M., Waters, E. and Wall, S. (1978). *Patterns of Attachment*. Hillsdale, NJ: Erlbaum.

Alderson, P. (1995). *Listening to Children*. Barkingside: Barnardos.

Aldgate, J. and Bradley, M. (1994). 'Short-term family based care for children in need', *Adoption and Fostering,* **18**, 4.

Aldridge, J. and Becker, S. (1994). *My Child My Carer – The Parent's Perspective*. Loughborough University, Loughborough, (Department of Social Sciences) in association with Nottingham Health Authority and Nottinghamshire Association of Voluntary Organisations, Nottingham.

Allen, S. and Morris, B. (1992). 'Oasis: the mental health in the community project'. In: B. Lynch and R. Perry (Eds) *Experiences of Community Care*. London: Longman.

AMA (1993). *Mental Health Services*. London: AMA.

Ammerman, R.T., van Hassels, V.B. and Hemem, M. (1988). 'Abuse and neglect in handicapped children: a critical review,' *Journal of Family Violence*, **3**, 53–72.

Anthony, E.J. (1986). 'Terrorising attacks on children by psychotic parents', *Journal of the American Academy of Child Psychiatry*, **25**, 326–335.

Apfel, R.J. and Handel, M.H. (1993). *Madness and Loss of Motherhood*. Washington: American Psychiatric Press.

Appleby, L. and Dickens, C. (1993). 'Mothering skills of women with mental illness'

Audit Commission (1994). *Finding a Place: a Review of Mental Health Services for Adults*. London: HMSO.

Audit Commission (1996). *Misspent Youth*. London: HMSO.

Ayalon, O. and Flasher, A. (1993). *Chain Reaction, Children and Divorce*. London: Jessica Kingsley.

Bainham, A. (1990). *Children, the New Law: The Children Act 1989*. London: Family Law.

Barham, P. (1992). *Closing the Asylum*. Harmondsworth: Penguin.

Barn, R. (1990). 'Black Children in Local Authority Care: Admission Patterns', *New Community,* **16**(2), 229–246.

Barn, R. (1993). *Black Children in the Public Care System*. Batsford: BAAF.

Barnardos (1992). *You Grow Up Fast as Well*. Barkingside: Barnardos.

Bayley, N. (1969). *Bayley Scales of Infant Development*. New York: Psychological Corporation.

Bell, J. (1995). *Doing Your Research Project*. Milton Keynes: Open University Press.

Belsky, J. and Rovine, M. (1988). 'Nonmaternal care in the first year of life and the security of infant-parent attachment', *Child Development,* **59**, 157–167.

Bernardi, S., Jones, M. and Tennant, C. (1989). 'Quality of parenting in alcoholics and narcotics addicts', *British Journal of Psychiatry,* **154**, 677–682.

Black, D. (1990). 'What do children need from parents?' *Early Child Development and Care,* **60**, 11–22.

Blanch, A.K., Nicholson, J. and Purcell, J. (1994). 'Parents with severe mental illness and their children: the need for human services integration', *Journal of Mental Health Administration,* **21**, 4.

Blom Cooper, L. (1992). *Report of the Committee of Inquiry into Complaints at Ashworth Hospital*. London: HMSO.

Blum, D. (1995). 'Early push to weed out unfit haunts the IQ field', *Sacramento Bee,* 15 October.

Boath, E.M., Barnett, B., Britto, D., Bryce, A. and Cox, J.L. (1995). 'When the bough breaks: Charles Street Parent and Baby Day Unit', *Journal of Reproductive and Infant Psychology,* **13**, 237–240.

Boath, E., Cox, J.L., Lewis, M. Jones, P. and Pryce, A. (in press). 'When the cradle falls: the treatment of PND in a psychiatric day hospital compared with routine primary care, *British Medical Journal*.

Bowlby, J. (1969). *Attachment and Loss. Vol.1: Attachment*. London: Hogarth Press.

Boyce, P. (1994). 'Personality dysfunction, marital problems and postnatal depression'. In: J.L. Cox and J. Holden (Eds) *Perinatal Psychiatry. Use and Misuse of the Edinburgh Postnatal Depression Scale*. London: Gaskell Press.

Brandon, A. and Brandon, D. (1987). *Consumers as Colleagues*. London: MIND Publications.

Brandon, D. (1981). *Voices of Experience – Consumer Perspectives of Psychiatric Treatment*. London: MIND Publications.

Brindle, D. (1996). 'Distress signals', *Guardian,* 10 July.

Brown, G. and Harris, T. (1976). *Social Origins of Depression. A Study of Psychiatric Disorders in Women.* London: Tavistock.

Brown, G. and Harris, T. (1978). *Social Origins of Depression.* London: Tavistock.

Brown, G.W. and Birley, J.L.T. (1968). 'Crises and life changes and the onset of schizophrenia', *Journal of Health and Social Behaviour,* **9**, 203–214.

Browne, K. and Lynch, M. (1995). 'Editorial', *Child Abuse Review,* **4,** 309–316.

Budd, K.S. and Holdsworth, M.J. (1996). 'Issues in clinical assessment of minimal parenting competence', *Journal of Clinical Child Psychology,* **25**, 2–14.

Burgess, R. (1984). *In the Field.* London: Allen and Unwin.

Caplan, P.J. (1995). *They Say You're Crazy. How The World's Most Powerful Psychiatrists Decide Who's Normal.* Reading, MA: Addison Wesley.

Caplan, H. *et al.* (1989). 'Maternal depression and the emotional development of the child', *British Journal of Psychiatry,* **154**, 818–822.

Carers National Association (1992). *Speak Up, Speak Out: Research Amongst Members of Carers National Association.* London: Carers National Association.

Carson, D. (1994). 'Dangerous people: through a broader concept of "risk" and "danger" to better decisions', *Expert Evidence,* **3**(2), 51–69.

CCETSW (1993). *Requirements and Guidance for the Training of Social Workers to be Considered for Approval in England and Wales under the Mental Health Act 1983.* London: CCETSW.

Chadwick, P. and Birchwood, M. (1994). 'The omnipotence of voices: A cognitive approach to auditory hallucinations', *British Journal of Psychiatry,* **164**, 190–201.

Cheetham, J., Fuller, R., McIvor, G. and Petch, A. (1994). *Evaluating Social Work Effectiveness.* Milton Keynes: Open University Press.

Chiswick, D. (1995). 'Dangerousness'. In: D. Chiswick and R. Cope (Eds) *Seminars in Practical Forensic Psychiatry.* London: Gaskell Press/Royal College of Psychiatrists.

Ciompi, L. (1980). 'The natural history of schizophrenia in the long-term', *British Journal of Psychiatry,* **136**, 413–420.

Clifford, C., Day, A. and Cox, J.L. (1997). 'Developing the use of EPDS in a Punjabi-speaking community,' *British Journal of Midwifery,* **5**(10), 616–619.

Clyde, J. (1992). *The Report of the Inquiry Into the Removal of Children from Orkney in February 1991.* London: HMSO.

Cogan, J. (1993). *Accessing the Community Support Service Needs Women with Psychiatric Disabilities may have Regarding Relationships.* Doctoral Dissertation. Vermont: Centre for Community Change.

Cohen, L. and Manion, L. (1994). *Research Methods in Education.* London: Routledge.

Commonwealth Department Human Services and Health (1994). *National Mental Project Funding Innovative Grants Programme.* Canberra: AGPS.

Cox, A.D. (1987). 'The impact of maternal depression on young children', *Journal of Child Psychology and Psychiatry,* **28**(6), 9–28.

Cox, A.D. (1988). 'Maternal depression and impact on children's development', *Archive of Disease in Childhood,* **63**, 90–95.

Cox, J.L. and Holden, J.M. (Eds) (1994). *Perinatal Psychiatry: Use and Misuse of the Edinburgh Postnatal Depression Scale*. London: Gaskell.

Cox, J.L., Gerrard, J., Cookson, D. and Jones, M.J. (1993). 'Development and audit of Charles Street Parent and Baby Day Unit, Stoke on Trent', *Psychiatric Bulletin*, **17**, 711–713.

Cox, J.L., Holden, J.M. and Sagovsky, R. (1987). 'Detection of postnatal depression; development of the Edinburgh Postnatal Depression Scale', *British Journal of Psychiatry*, **150**, 766–782.

Crittenden, P. and Clausen, H. (1993). 'Severity of maltreatment: assessment and policy implications'. In: C. Hobbs and J. Wynne (Eds) *Clinical Paediatrics: Child Abuse*. London: Ballière Tindall, pp. 87–101.

Cross-National Collaborative Group (1992). 'The changing rate of major depression Cross-national comparisons', *Journal of the American Medical Association*, **268**(21), 3098–3105.

Cummings, E.M. and Davies, P.T. (1994). 'Maternal depression and child development', *Journal of Child Psychology and Psychiatry*, **35**, 73–112.

Dale, P. with Davies, M., Morrison, T. and Waters, J. (1986). *Dangerous Families*. London: Tavistock Publications.

Darton, K., Gorman, J. and Sayce, L. (1994). *Eve Fights Back*. London: MIND Publications.

David, H.P. and Morgall, J.M. (1990). 'Family planning for the mentally disordered and retarded', *Journal of Nervous and Mental Disease*, **178**, 385–391.

Deardon, C. and Becker, S. (1995). *Young Carers, the Facts*. Community Care, Reed Business Publishing/Young Carers Research Group.

Department of Health (1983). *The Mental Health Act 1983*. London: HMSO.

Department of Health (1989). *The Children Act 1989*. London: HMSO.

Department of Health (1990a). *The Care Programme Approach for people with a mental illness referred to the specialist psychiatric services*. HC(90)23, LASSL(90)11.

Department of Health (1990b). *NHS and Community Care Act 1990*. London: HMSO.

Department of Health (1991). *Working Together Under the Children Act 1989: A Guide to Arrangements for Inter-agency Co-operation for the Protection of Children from Abuse*. London: HMSO.

Department of Health (1995a). *The Challenge of Partnership in Child Protection: Practice Guide*. London: HMSO.

Department of Health (1995b). *Child Protection: Messages from Research*. London: HMSO.

Department of Health (1995c). *Child Health in the Community: A Guide to Good Practice*. London: Department of Health, p. 55.

Department of Health (1995d). *Mental Health Patients in the Community Act 1995*. London: HMSO.

Department of Health (1996a). *Building Bridges – A Guide to Arrangements for Inter-agency Working for the Care and Protection of Severely Mentally Ill People*. London: HMSO, p. 41.

Department of Health (1996b). *Children's Services Planning: Guidance*. London: Department of Health.

Department of Health (1996c). *The Carers Services and Recognition Act 1996*. London: HMSO.

Department of Health (1998). *Crossing Bridges: Training Resources for Working with Mentally Ill Parents and Their Children*. London: HMSO.

Desjarlais, R., Eisenberg, L., Good, B. and Kleinman, A. (1995). *World Mental Health: Problems and Priorities in Low Income Countries*. Oxford: Oxford University Press.

Disability Compliance Bulletin (1996). Horsham, PA, USA: LRP Publications.

Doleman, D. (1987). 'Thriving despite hardship: Key childhood traits identified', *New York Times*, 13 October.

Dominian, J. (1968). *Marital Breakdown*. London: Penguin.

Dowdney, L. and Skuse, D. (1993). 'Parenting provided by adults with mental retardation', *Journal of Child Psychology and Psychiatry*, **34**, 25–47.

Dwivedi, K.N. (1996). 'Culture and personality'. In: K.N. Dwivedi and V.P. Varma (Eds) *Meeting the Needs of Ethnic Minority Children*. London: Jessica Kingsley, pp. 17–33.

Elliott, A. (1992). *Hidden Children – A Study of Ex-young Carers of Parents with Mental Health Problems in Leeds*. Leeds: Leeds City Council Social Services Department.

Evans, M. and Miller, C. (1995). *Joint Commissioning for Child Protection – A Future Role for Area Child Protection Committees?* London: Office for Public Management.

Fadden, G., Bebbington, P. and Kuipers, L. (1987). 'The burden of care: impact of functional psychiatric illness on the patient's family', *British Journal of Psychiatry*, **150**, 285–292.

Falkov, A. (1995). *Troubled Lives: Psychiatric Morbidity in Children Living with Psychotic Parents*. London: Department of Child and Family Psychiatry, UMDS and West Lambeth.

Falkov, A. (1996). *Working Together, Part 8: Reports, Fatal Child Abuse and Parental Psychiatric Disorder*. London: Department of Health.

Falkov, A. (1997). *Parental Psychiatric Disorder and Child Maltreatment. Parts I and II*, National Children's Bureau, Highlight Series No. 149, January 1997.

Feldman, R.A., Stiffman, A.R. and Jung, K.G. (1987). *Children at Risk: in the Web of Parental Mental Illness*. New Brunswick: Rutgers University Press.

Field, I.M. (1993). 'Enhancing parent sensitivity'. In: N.J. Anastasion and S. Harel (Eds) *At Risk Infants: Interventions, Families and Research*. Baltimore: Paul H. Brooks Publishing Co., pp. 81–89.

Fisher, M., Newton, C. and Sainsbury, E. (1984). *Mental Health Social Work Observed*. London: Allen and Unwin.

Fitzgerald, M.H. (1995). 'Cultural breaks in women's knowledge'. In: Marce Pacific Rim Conference: Childbearing and Mental Health – Risk and Remedies. Marce Society presentation, Sydney, Australia.

Frank, J. (1995). *Couldn't Care More – A Study of Young Carers and Their Needs*. London: The Children's Society.

Garmezy, N., Masten, A.S. and Tellegen, A. (1984). 'The study of stress and competence in children: a building block for developmental psychopathology', *Child Development*, **55**, 97–111.

Gath, A. (1988). 'Mentally handicapped people as parents', *Journal of Child Psychology and Psychiatry*, **29**, 739–744.

George, M. (1992). 'Sacrificing children on the altar of care', *Community Care*, 11 June, 27–28.

Gillberg, C. and Geijer-Karlsson, M. (1983). 'Children born to mentally retarded women: A 1–21 year follow-up study of 41 cases', *Psychological Medicine*, **13**, 891–894.

Golden, (1991). 'Do the Disability Rights and Right-to-life movements have any common ground? *Disability Rag*, **9**, 91.

Goldstein, M. (1987). 'Psychosocial issues', *Schizophrenia Bulletin*, **13**, 157–171.

Gooding, C. (1995). *Blackstone's Guide to the Disability Discrimination Act*. London: Blackstone Press.

Goodman, S. (1984). 'Children of disturbed parents: the interface between research and intervention', *American Journal of Community Psychology*, **12**, 663–687.

Goodman, S.H. and Brumley, H.E. (1990). 'Schizophrenic and depressed mothers: Relational deficits in parenting', *Developmental Psychology*, **26**, 31–39.

Goodyear, L. (1990). 'Family relationships, life events and childhood psychopathology', *Journal of Child Psychology and Psychiatry*, **31**(1), 161–192.

Gopfert, M., Webster, J., Pollard, J. and Nelki, J.S. (1996). 'The assessment and prediction of parenting capacity: A community-oriented approach'. In: M. Gopfert, J. Webster and M.V. Seeman (Eds) *Parental Psychiatric Disorder: Distressed Parents and their Children*. Cambridge: Cambridge University Press.

Gorman, J. (1992). *Out of the Shadows*. London: MIND Publications.

Gostin, L.O. (1993). 'Genetic discrimination in employment and insurance'. In: L.O. Gostin and H.A. Beyer (Eds) *Implementing the Americans with Disabilities Act*. Baltimore: Paul H. Brookes Publishing Co.

Gottesman, L.L. (1991). *Schizophrenia Genesis*. New York: Freeman.

Gould, S.J. (1985). *The Flamingo's Smile*. New York and London: W.H. Norton and Co.

Hagnell, O., Lanke, J., Rorsman, B. and Ojeso, L. (1982). 'Are we entering an age of Melancholy? Depressive illnesses in a prospective epidemiological study over 25 years: the Lundby Study, Sweden,' *Journal of Psychological Medicine*, **12**(2), 279–289.

Hall, A. (1996). 'Parental psychiatric disorder and the developing child'. In: M. Gopfert, J. Webster and M.V. Seeman (Eds) *Parental Psychiatric Disorder: Distressed Parents and their Children*. Cambridge: Cambridge University Press.

Hammen, C. (1993). 'The family – environmental context of depression'. In: D. Cicchetti and S. Toth (Eds) *Rochester Symposium on Developmental Psychopathology*, Vol. 4. Hillsdale, NJ: Erlbaum.

Hargreaves, R.G. and Hadlow, J. (1995). 'Preventative intervention as a working concept in childcare practice', *British Journal of Social Work*, **25**(3), 349–365.

Hawton, K. (1981). 'The association between child abuse and attempted suicide', *British Journal of Social Work*, **11**(4), 415–420.

*ꞇ*Heal, S. (1993). *Young Carers and the Children Act 1989*. London: Carers National Association.

Health Advisory Service (1995). *Child and Adolescent Mental Health Services*. London: HMSO, p. 2.

*ꞩ*Herbert, M. (1996). *Assessing Children in Need and Their Parents*. Leicester: BPS Books (The British Psychological Society).

Hill, J. (1996). 'Parental psychiatric disorder and the attachment relationship'. In: M. Gopfert, J. Webster and M.V. Seeman (Eds) *Parental Psychiatric Disorder: Distressed Parents and their Children*. Cambridge: Cambridge University Press.

Hipwell, A.E. and Kumar, R. (1996). 'Maternal psychopathology and prediction of outcome based on mother–infant interaction ratings (BMIS)', *British Journal of Psychiatry*, **169**, 655–661.

Hodges, J. and Tizard, B. (1989). 'IQ and behavioral adjustment of ex-institutional adolescents', *Journal of Child Psychology and Psychiatry*, **30**, 53–75, 77–98.

Hudson, B. (1982). *Social Work with Psychiatric Patients*. London: Macmillan.

Hughes, B. and Logan, J. (1995). 'The agenda for post-adoption services', *Adoption and Fostering*, **19**, 1.

Hugman, R. and Phillips, N. (1993). 'Like bees around the honeypot – social work responses to parents with mental health needs', *Practice* **6**(3), 193–205.

Hunter Johnston, E. (1996) Letter from Head of Children's Services Branch, Department of Health, to ACPC Chairs. 21 February.

Isaac, B., Minty, E. and Morrison, R. (1986a). 'Children in care – the association with mental disorder in the parents', *British Journal of Social Work*, **16**, 325–339.

Isaac, B., Minty, E. and Morrison, R. (1986b). 'Children in care : the association with mental disorder in parents', *Social Work and Social Sciences Review*, **4**(1), 27–58.

Jamison, K.R. (1995). *An Unquiet Mind. A Memoir of Moods and Madness*. New York: Alfred A Knopf.

Jenkins, S. and Wingate, C. (1994). 'Who cares for young carers?' *British Medical Journal*, **308**, 733–734.

Jones, R. (1994). *Mental Health Act Manual*. Andover: Sweet and Maxwell

Junginger, J. (1990). 'Predicting compliance with command hallucinations', *American Journal of Psychiatry*, **147**(2), 245–247.

Junginger, J. (1995). 'Command hallucinations and prediction of dangerousness', *Psychiatric Services*, **46**(9), 911–914.

Junginger, J., Barker, S. and Coe, D. (1992). 'Mood theme and bizarreness of delusions in schizophrenia and mood psychosis', *Journal of Abnormal Psychology*, **101**(2), 287–292.

Kendell, R.E., Chalmers, L. and Platz, C. (1987). 'The epidemiology of puerperal psychoses', *British Journal of Psychiatry*, **150**, 622–673.

King, J. (1988). 'Working with child abusers – Setting the scene', *Community Care*, 29 April (Supplement).

Kolvin, I., Miller, F.J.W., Fleeting, M. and Kolvin, P.A. (1988). 'Social and parenting factors affecting criminal offence rates', *British Journal of Psychiatry*, **152**, 80–90.

Koreen, A.R., Siris, S.G., Chakos, M., Alvir, J., Mayerhoff, D. and Lieberman, J. (1993). 'Depression in first-episode schizophrenia', *American Journal of Psychiatry*, **150**(11), 1643–1648.

Kumar, R.C. and Hipwell, A.I.E. (1994). 'Implications for the infant of maternal puerperal psychiatric disorders'. In: M. Rutter, E.A. Taylor and L.A. Hersov (Eds) *Child and Adolescent Psychiatry: Modern Approaches*. Oxford: Blackwell Scientific Publications.

Kumar, R., Marks, M., Platz, C. and Yoshida, K. (1995). 'Clinical survey of a psychiatric mother and baby unit: Characteristics of 100 consecutive admissions', *Journal of Affective Disorders*, **33**, 11–22.

Laming, H. (1995/6). *Progress Through Change: The 5th Annual Report of the Chief Inspector of Social Services, Department of Health*. London: HMSO.

Lau, A. (1991). 'Cultural and ethnic perspectives on significant harm: Its assessment and treatment'. In: M. Adcock, R. White, and A. Hollows (Eds) *Significant Harm: Its Management and Outcome*. Croydon: Significant Publications.

Lau, A. (1995). 'Gender, power and relationships; ethnocultural and religious issues'. In: C. Burck, and B. Speed (Eds) *Gender, Power and Relationships*. London: Routledge.

Laxova, R., Gilderdale, S. and Ridler, M.A.C. (1973). 'An aetiological study of fifty-three female patients from a subnormality hospital and of their offspring', *Journal of Mental Deficiency Research*, **17**, 193–217.

Lee, F. (1996). 'The great paper chase', *Community Care*, 20 June.

Leighton Cox, D. (1988). 'Being mentally ill in America: One female experience'. In: L.L. Bachrach and C.C. Nadelson (Eds) *Treating Chronically Mentally Ill Women*. Washington DC: American Psychiatric Press.

Lewis, A.J. (1956). 'Lecture on the scientific basis of medicine', *Social Psychiatry*, **VI** (1957–7), 116.

Link, B.G. and Stueve, A. (1994). 'Psychotic symptoms and the violent/illegal behaviour of mental patients compared to community controls'. In: J. Monahan and H.J. Steadman (Eds) *Violence and Mental Disorder: Developments in Risk Assessment*. Chicago: University of Chicago Press, pp. 137–159.

Link, B.G., Andrews, H. and Cullen, F.T. (1992). 'Reconsidering the violent and illegal behaviour of mental patients', *American Sociological Review*, **57**, 275–292.

Lombardo, P. (1983). 'Involuntary sterilisation in Virginia: From Buck v Bell to Poe v Lynchburg', *Developments in Mental Health Law*, **3**(3).

Lombardo, P. (1985). 'Three generations, no imbeciles: New light on Buck v Bell', *New York University Law Review*, **60**(1).

Londerville, S. and Main, M. (1981). 'Security of attachment, compliance, and maternal training methods in the second year of life', *Developmental Psychology*, **17**, 289–299.

Maher, B.A. (1988). 'Anomalous experience and delusional thinking: the logic of explanations'. In: T.F. Oltmanns and B.A. Maher (Eds) *Delusional Beliefs*. New York: Wiley.

Manchester University and the Department of Health (1996). *Learning Materials on Mental Health*.

Mancuso, L.L. (1993). *Case Studies on Reasonable Accommodation for Workers with Psychiatric Disabilities*. California: Centre for Mental Health Services and California Department of Mental Health.

Manic Depression Fellowship (1992). *Parenthood and Manic Depressive Illness*. London: Manic Depression Fellowship Limited.

Mapp, S. (1994). 'Looking out for mother's help', *Community Care*, 8 June.

Marks, M.N. and Kumar, F.T. (1995). 'Infanticide in England and Wales 1982–1988', *Medicine, Science and the Law,* **33**, 329–339.

Marsh, P. and Triseolitis, J. (1996). *Ready to Practice? Social Workers and Probation Officers: Their Training and First Year in Work*. Aldershot: Avebury Press.

McCall, R.B. (1983). 'A conceptual approach to early mental development'. In: M. Lewis (Ed.) *Origins of Intelligence: Infancy and Early Childhood*. New York: Plenum.

McGorry, P.D., Chanen, A., McCarthy, E., Van Riel, R., McKenzie, D. and Singh, B. (1991). 'Post-traumatic Stress Disorder following recent-onset psychosis', *Journal of Nervous and Mental Disease*, **179**(5), 253–258.

McGuffin, P., Owen, M.J. and Farmer, A.E. (1995). 'Genetic basis of schizophrenia', *Lancet*, **346**, September 9.

Mental Health Act Commission (1993). *Fifth Biennial Report*. London: HMSO.

Mental Health Association in New York State (1996) *Parents with Psychiatric Disabilities Support Project Mental Health: Problems and Priorities in Low Income Countries*. Oxford: Oxford University Press.

Miles, C.P. (1977). 'Conditions pre-disposing to suicide: A review', *Journal of Nervous and Mental Disease,* **164**, 231–246.

Miller, L.J. (1992). 'Comprehensive care of pregnant mentally ill women', *Journal of Mental Health Administration* **19**, 2.

Milner, J. (1995). 'Physical child abuse assessment: perpetrator evaluation'. In: J. Campbell (Ed.) *Assessing Dangerousness: Violence by Sexual Offenders, Batterers and Child Abusers*. London: Sage.

MIND (1992). *Stress on Women Pack*. London: MIND.

MIND (1993). *MIND's Policy on Women and Mental Health*. London: MIND.

MIND (1996). *Journal of Community Care*, **22**.

Mino, Y. and Ushijima, S. (1989). 'Postpsychotic collapse in schizophrenia', *Acta Psychiatric. Scand.*, **80**, 368–374.

Mowbray, C.T. and Benedek, E.P. (1990). *Women's Mental Health Research Agenda: Services and Treatments of Mental Disorders in Women*. Occasional Paper, US Department of Health and Human Services.

Mowbray, C.T., Oyersman, D., Zemencuk, J.K. and Ross, S.R. (1995). 'Motherhood for women with serious mental illness', *American Journal of Orthopsychiatry,* **65**(1).

Mrazek, D.A., Mrazek, P. and Kimnert, M. (1995). 'Clinical assessment of parenting', *Journal of the American Academy of Child and Adolescent Psychiatry*, **34**, 272–282.

Mulvey, E.P. (1994). 'Assessing the evidence of a link between mental illness and violence', *Hospital and Community Psychiatry*, **45**(7), 663–668.

Murray L. and Stein, A. (1989). 'The effects of postnatal depression on mother–infant relations and infant development'. In: N. Woodhead, R. Carr and P. Light (Eds) *Becoming a Person*. London: Routledge.

Murray, D., Cox, J.L., Chapman, G. and Jones, P. (1995). 'Childbirth: Life event or start of a long term difficulty? Further data from the Stoke on Trent Controlled Study of Postnatal Depression', *British Journal of Psychiatry*, **166**, 595–600.

Murray, L. (1992). 'The impact of postnatal depression on infant development', *Journal of Child Psychology and Psychiatry*, **33**, 543–561.

Murray, L. and Trevarthen, C. (1985). 'Emotional regulation of interactions between 2-month-olds and their mothers'. In: T.M. Field and N.A. Fox (Eds) *Social Perception in Infants*. Norwood, NJ: Ablex

Murray, L., Hipwell, A., Hooper, R., Stein, A. and Cooper, P. (1996). 'The cognitive development of 5-year-old children of postnatally depressed mothers', *Journal of Child Psychology and Psychiatry*, **37**, 927–935.

NAMI (1996). *Summary of Highlights from a National Public Opinion Survey of Americans' Awareness and Attitudes Regarding Serious Brain Disorders*. Arlington, VA: National Alliance for the Mentally Ill.

Neuberger, J. (1994). 'Commentary: Year of the family', *Journal of the Royal Society of Arts*, July, p. 4.

New South Wales (1994). *New South Wales: Postnatal Depression Services Review*. State Health Publication No. (PA) 94–131.

Newton, J. (1988). *Preventing Mental Illness*. London: Routledge.

Nicholson, J. and Blanch, A. (1994). 'Rehabilitation for parenting roles for people with serious mental illness', *Psychosocial Rehabilitation Journal*, **18**, 1.

Nicholson, J., Geller, J.L., Fisher, W.H. and Dion, G.L. (1993). 'State programmes and policies that address the needs of mentally ill mothers in the public sector', *Hospital and Community Psychiatry*, **44**(5).

Nicholson, J., Geller, J.L. and Fisher, W.H. (1996). 'A case study for policy makers: Sylvia Frumkin has a baby', *Psychiatric Services*, **47**(5).

'No ADA Violation in Parental Rights Case' (1996).*World Disability Compliance Bulletin* **6**(8) 11 May.

Northumbria Probation Service Sex Offenders Team and the Department of Adolescent Forensic Psychiatry, Newcastle Mental Health Trust (1994). 'Learning from perpetrators of child sexual abuse', *Probation Journal*, September, 147–151.

NSPCC (1997). *Long-Term Problems . . . Short Term Solutions*. London: NSPCC Practice Development Unit.

Oakley, A., Mauthney, M., Rajan, L. and Turner, H. (1995). 'Supporting vulnerable families: an evaluation of Newpin', *Health Visitor*, **68**(5), 188.

Office of Population Censuses and Surveys (1995). *Psychiatric Morbidity among Adults in Great Britain. Report on the Prevalence of Psychiatric Morbidity among Adults Living in Private Households*. London: OPCS.

O'Hara, M.W. and Zekoski, E.M. (1988). 'Postpartum depression: a comprehensive review'. In: R. Kumar and I.F. Brockington (Eds) *Motherhood and Mental Illness*, Vol. 2. London: Wright.

Oyersman, D., Mowbray, C.T. and Zemencuk, J.K. (1992). 'Mothers with a severe mental illness: What does the past decade of research show?' *British Journal of Social Work*, **6**, 815–845.

Penfold, S. and Walker, G. (1984). *Women and the Psychiatric Paradox*. Milton Keynes: Open University Press.

Perkins, R. (1992). 'Catherine is having a baby', *Feminism and Psychology*, **2**(1), 110–112.

Phillips, A. (1994). 'Out in MIND', *Openmind*, 68.

Pitt, B. (1968). '"Atypical" depression following childbirth', *British Journal of Psychiatry*, **114**, 1325–1335.

Poole, R. (1996). 'General adult psychiatrists and their patients' children'. In: M. Gopfert, J. Webster and M. V. Seeman (Eds) *Parental Psychiatric Disorder: Distressed Parents and their Families*. Cambridge: Cambridge University Press.

Prettyman, R.J. and Friedman, T. (1991). 'Care of women with puerperal psychiatric disorder in England and Wales', *British Medical Journal*, **302**, 1345–1346.

Price, C.R. (1995). 'Determinants in motherhood in human and non-human primates: a biosocial model'. In: *Determinants of Motherhood in Human and Non-human Primates*. Basle: Karger.

Puckering, C. (1989). 'Annotation: Maternal depression', *Journal of Child Psychology and Psychiatry*, **126**, 325–334.

Quinton, D. and Rutter, M. (1984). 'Parents with children in care', *Psychology and Psychiatry*, **25**, 211–229

Ramsay, R. and Kumar, C. (1996). 'Ethical dilemmas in perinatal psychiatry', *Psychiatric Bulletin*, **20**, 90–92.

Reed, E.W. and Reed, S.C. (1965). *Mental Retardation: A Family Study*. Philadelphia: W.B. Saunders.

Reed, J. and Baker, S. (1996). *Not Just Sticks and Stones*. London: MIND.

Reich, W., Earls, F., Frankel, O. and Shayka, J. (1993). 'Psychopathology in children and adolescents', *Journal of the American Academy of Child and Adolescent Psychiatry*, **32**(5), 995–1002.

Release (1995). *Women and Drugs*. London: Release Publications.

Report of the Inquiry into Child Abuse in Cleveland (1987). London: HMSO.

Report of the Inquiry into the Treatment and Care of Darren Carr (1997). Oxford: Oxfordshire District Health Authority.

Report of the Panel of Inquiry Presented to the Tees District Health Authority into the Treatment and Care of Sean Armstrong (1996). Middlesborough: Tees District Health Authority.

Repper, J. and Brooker, C. (1996). *A Review of Public Attitudes Towards Mental Health Facilities in the Community*. Sheffield Centre for Health and Related Research.

Reynolds, C.R. and Kamphaus, R.W. (1992). *Behaviour Assessment System for Children*. Circle Pines: American Guidance Service.

Richman, N. (1977). 'Behaviour problems in pre-school children: family and social factors', *British Journal of Psychiatry*, **131**, 523–527.

Richman, N., Stevenson J. and Graham, P.J. (1982). *Preschool to School: A Behavioural Study*. London: Academic Press.

Rickford, F. (1996a). 'Mum needs me', *Guardian Society*, 7 December, pp. 6–7.

Rickford, F. (1996b). 'The ties that bind'. *Community Care*, 6 June.

Rimpoche, D.A. (1987). *Taming the Tiger*. Eskdalemuir: Dzalendra Publishing.

Ritchie, J., Dick, D., Lingham, R. (1994). *Report of the Inquiry into the Care and Treatment of Christopher Clunis*. London: HMSO.

Ritsner, J.E., Karas, S.I. and Drigalenko, E.I. (1991). 'Genetic epidemiological study of schizophrenia: two modes of sampling', *Genetic Epidemiology*, **8**, 47–53.

Robins, L.N. and Regier, D.A. (Eds) (1991). *Psychiatric Disorders in America*. New York: The Free Press.

Rogers, A., Pilgrim, D. and Lacey, R. (1990). *Experiencing Psychiatry*. London: MIND.

Rogosh, R.A., Mowbray, C.T. and Bogat, G.A. (1992). 'Determinants of parenting attitudes in mothers with severe psychopathology', *Development and Psychopathology*, **4**, 469–487.

Rosenfield, S. (1989). 'The effect of women's employment: Personal control and sex differences in mental health', *Journal of Health and Social Behaviour*, **30**, 77–91.

Roy, R. (1990/1). 'Consequences of parental illness on children: A review', *Social Work and Social Sciences Review*, **2**(2), 109–121.

Royal College of Psychiatrists (1992). *Working Party Report on Postnatal Mental Illness*. Council Report CR28, London: Royal College of Psychiatrists.

Royal College of Psychiatrists (1996). *Confidential Inquiry into Homicides and Suicides by Mentally Ill People*. London: Royal College of Psychiatrists.

Rubenstein, L.S. (1993). 'Mental disorder and the ADA'. In: L.O. Gostin and H.A. Beyer (Eds) *Implementing the Americans with Disabilities Act*. Baltimore: Paul H. Brookes Publishing Co.

Rutter, M. (1990). 'Commentary – some focus and process considerations regarding effects of parental depression on children', *Developmental Psychology*, **26**, 60–67.

Rutter, M. (1982). 'Epidemiological–longitudinal approaches to the study of development'. In: W.A. Collins, (Ed.) *The Concept of Development, Minnesota Symposia on Child Psychology*, Vol. 15. Hillsdale, NJ: Erlbaum, pp 105–144.

Rutter, M. and Quinton, D. (1984). 'Parental psychiatric disorder: effects on children', *Psychological Medicine*, **14**, 853–880.

Rutter, M. and Quinton, D. (1987). 'Parental mental illness as a risk factor for psychiatric disorder in childhood'. In: D. Magnusson and A. Ohman (Eds) *Psychopathology: An Interactional Perspective*. Orlando, FL: Academic Press.

Rutter, M., MacDonald, H., LeCouteur, A., Harrington, R., Bolton, P. and Bailey, A. (1990). 'Genetic factors in child psychiatric disorders, empirical findings', *Journal of Child Psychology and Psychiatry*, **31**, 39–83.

Rynearson, E.K. (1982). 'Relinquishment and its maternal complications: A preliminary study', *American Journal of Psychiatry*, **139**, 338–340.

Sackett, R.S. (1991). 'Terminating parental rights of the handicapped', *Family Law Quarterly*, **25**(3).

Sameroff, A.J. and Seifer, R. (1990). 'Early contributions to developmental risk'. In: J. Rolf, A.S. Mastern, D. Cicchetti, K.H. Nueehterlein and S. Weintraub (Eds), *Risk and Protective Factors in Development of Psychopathology*. Cambridge: Cambridge University Press.

Sands, R. G. (1995). 'The parenting experience of low-income single women with serious mental disorders – families and society', *The Journal of Comtemporary Human Services*, pp.86–96.

Saunders, A. (1995). *'It hurts me too', Children's Experiences of Domestic Violence and Refuge Life*. WAFE, NISW, Childline.

Sayce, L. (1995). 'Response to violence: A framework for fair treatment'. In: J. Crichton (Ed.) *Psychiatric Patient Violence*. London: Duckworth.

Sayce, L. (1996). 'Women with Children'. In: R. Perkins (Ed.) *Women in Context*. London: Good Practices in Mental Health.

Schaffer, H.R. and Emerson, P.E. (1964). 'The development of social attachments in infancy', *Monographs of the Society for Research in Child Development*, **29** (3, Serial no.94).

Schuff, G.H. and Asen, K.E. (1996). 'The disturbed parent and the disturbed family'. In: M. Gopfert, J. Webster and M.V. Seeman (Eds) *Parental Psychiatric Disorder*. Cambridge: Cambridge University Press, pp. 135–151.

Seeman, M.V. (1996). 'The mother with schizophrenia'. In: M. Gopfert, J. Webster and M.V Seeman (Eds) *Parental Psychiatric Disorder: Distressed Parents and their Children*. Cambridge: Cambridge University Press.

Sheppard, M. (1993). 'The external context for social support : towards a theoretical formulation of social support, child care and maternal depression', *Social Work and Social Sciences Review*, **4**(1), 27–58.

Sheppard, M. (1994). 'Maternal depression. Child care and the social work role', *British Journal of Social Work*, **24**(1), 33–51.

Sheppard, M. (1997). 'The Psychiatric Unit'. In: Davies, M. (Ed.) *The Blackwell Companion to Social Work*. Oxford: Blackwell, pp. 317–323.

Sieff Foundation (1997). *Keeping Children in Mind*, (conference report). Sieff Foundation.

Silverman, M.M. (1989). 'Children of psychiatrically ill parents: a prevention perspective', *Hospital and Community Psychiatry*, **40**, 1257–1265.

Siris, S.G. (1991). 'Diagnosis of secondary depression in schizophrenia: implications for DSM-IV', *Schizophrenia Bulletin*, **17**(1), 75–98.

Slade, A. (1987). 'Quality of attachment and symbolic play', *Developmental Psychology*, **23**, 78–85.

Smith, S.M., Hanson, R. and Noble, S. (1973). 'Parents of battered babies: a controlled study', *British Medical Journal*, **4**, 388–391.

Starkey, A. (1996). *Marriage and the Modern Crisis; Repairing Married Life*. London: Hodder and Stoughton.

Sroufe, L.A., Fox, N.E. and Pancake, V.R. (1983). 'Attachment and dependency in developmental perspective', *Child Development*, **54**, 1615–1627.

Stefan, S. (1989). 'Whose egg is it anyway? Reproductive rights of incarcerated, institutionalised and incompetent women', *Nova Law Review,* **13**(2).

Steinhausen, H.C., Willms, J.and Spohr, H.L. (1993). 'Long term psychopathological and cognitive outcome of children with Fetal Alcohol Syndrome', *Journal of the American Academy of Child and Adolescent Psychiatry,* **32**(5), 990–994.

Stiffman, A., Jung, K. and Feldman, A. (1988). 'Parental mental illness, family living arrangements and child behaviour', *Journal of Social Service Research*, **11**(23), 21–34.

Strauss, M. A., Gelles, R.J. and Steinmetz, S.K. (1980). *Behind Closed Doors: Violence in the American Family*. Anchor/Doubleday.

Sutton, P. (1995). 'Built for the future', *Community Care,* 7 December, 16–17.

Swanson, J.W., Holzer, C.E., Ganju, V.K. *et al.* (1994). 'Violence and psychiatric disorder in the community: evidence from the epidemiological catchment area surveys', *Hospital and Community Psychiatry,* **41**, 761–770.

Taylor, C. *et al.* (1991). 'Diagnosed intellectual and emotional impairment among parents who seriously mistreat their children: prevalence, type and outcome in a court sample', *Child Abuse and Neglect,* **15**, 389–401.

Thomas, A. and Chess, S. (1977). *Temperament and Development.* New York: Brunner/Mazel.

Thompson, A. (1995). 'Special delivery', *Community Care,* 9 March.

Thompson, N. (1992). *Anti-Discriminatory Practice.* Basingstoke/Birmingham: BASW, Macmillan Press.

Thorburn, J., Lewis, J. and Shemmings, D. (1995). *Paternalism or Partnership? Family Involvement in the Child Protection Process.* London: HMSO.

Thorpe, D. (1994). *Evaluating Child Protection.* Buckingham: Open University Press.

Tizard, B. and Rees, J. (1974). 'A comparison of the effects of adoption, restoration to the natural mother and continued institutionalization on the cognitive development of four-year old children', *Child Development,* **45**, 92–99.

Toolis, K. (1998). 'Of human darkness', *Guardian Weekend,* 17 January.

Tymchuk, A.J. (1992). 'Predicting adequacy of parenting by people with mental retardation', *Child Abuse and Neglect,* **16**, 165–178.

Tymchuk, A.J., Yokota, A. and Rahbar, B. (1990). 'Decision-making abilities of mothers with mental retardation', *Research in Developmental Disabilities,* **11**, 97–109.

United Nations (1991). *Convention on the Rights of the Child.* New York: United Nations.

United Nations (1994). *International Year of the Family Pamphlet.* Vienna: United Nations.

United States Holocaust Memorial Museum (1996). *Handicapped.* Washington DC: United States Holocaust Memorial Museum.

Ussher, J.H. (1991). *Women's Madness: Misogyny or Mental Illness?* Harvester, Wheatsheaf.

Wang, A. R. and Goldschmidt, V.V. (1994). 'Interviews of psychiatric inpatients about the family situation and young children', *Acta Psychiatrica Scandinavica,* **90**, 459–465.

Warner, L. and Ford, R. (1996). 'Private investigation', *Health Service Journal*, April, 28–30.

Webster, J. (1992). 'Split in two: Experiences of the children of schizophrenic mothers', *British Journal of Social Work,* **22**(3), 309–329.

Webster, J. (1990). 'Parenting for children of schizophrenic mothers', *Adoption and Fostering,* **14**(2), 37–43.

Weintraubs, S. (1987). 'Risk factors in schizophrenia: the Stony Brook high risk project', *Schizophrenia Bulletin,* **13**, 439–449.

Weir, A. (1994). 'Split decisions', *Community Care*, July, 18.

Weissman, H. M., Leaf, P.J., Tischler, G.I., Blazer, D.G., Karno, M., Bruce, M.L. and Florio, L.P. (1988). 'Affective disorders in five United States countries', *Psychological Medicine,* **18**, 141–153.

Weissman, M.M., Paykel, E.S. (1974). *The Depressed Women*. University of Chicago.

Werner, E.E. (1986). 'Resilient offspring of alcoholics: A longitudinal study from birth to age 18', *Journal of Studies on Alcohol*, **47**, 34–40.

Whipple, E. and Webster-Stratton, C. (1991). 'The role of parental stress in physically abusive families', *Child Abuse and Neglect*, **15**, 279–291.

Williams, J. *et al.* (1993). *Purchasing Effective Services for Women*. Canterbury: University of Kent.

Williams, R. (1992). *A Concise Guide to the Children Act 1989*. London: Gaskell.

Wirral Health and Metropolitan Borough of Wirral (1995). *A Strategy for Wirral – Better Care for People with Mental Health Problems*. Birkenhead: Wirral Health Authority.

Women Against Rape and Legal Action for Women (1995). *Dossier: The Crime Prosecution Service and the Crime of Rape*. London: Women Against Rape.

Woodley Inquiry Team (1995). *Report of the Independent Review Panel to East London and the City Health Authority and Newham Council*. London: East London and the City Health Authority.

Zeanah, C.H., Boris, N.W. and Scheeringa, M.S. (1997). 'Psychopathology in infancy', *Journal of Child Psychology and Psychiatry*, **38**, 81–99.

Zeitlin, H. (1986). *The Natural History of Disorder in Childhood*. Institute of Psychiatry/Maudsley Monograph No. 29. Oxford: Oxford University Press.

Zeitz, M.A. (1995). 'The Mothers' Project: A clinical case management system', *Psychiatric Rehabilitation Journal*, **19**, 1.

Zito Trust (1995). *Learning the Lessons. Mental Health Inquiry Reports Published in England and Wales between 1969 and 1994 and their Recommendations for Improving Practice*. London: The Zito Trust.

Zubin, J. and Spring, B. (1977). 'Vulnerability: A new view of schizophrenia', *Journal of Abnormal Psychology*, **86**, 102–126.

Index

Abortion, 38, 40–1
Accreditation of social workers, 123
Adolescent socialization, 80–1
Adult psychiatrist's role, 17–22, 23–7
  child protection process, 26–7
  family interventions, 27
  lack of child-oriented facilities, 24–5, 106
  parenting capacity assessment, 24–5
Adventure Weekend Breaks Project, 139–40
Aggressive behaviour, 2, 18, 35
  see also Fatal child abuse; Physical abuse
Alcohol misuse, 4, 14, 20, 35
Americans with Disabilites Act (1990), 33, 35, 36, 37
Anti-discrimination principles, 32–4, 141
Antisocial personality disorders
  co-morbidity, 14
  predisposing factors in childhood, 90
Anxiety disorders, 2
  impact on children, 26
Assistance in coping, 4–5, 20
Association for Postnatal Illness
  volunteer register, 156
Attachment relationships, 54–5, 75, 89, 90

Australia, 5
  Early Psychosis Research Centre Project, 163–72
    aims, 165
    child carer problems, 166, 168
    family disruption, 167–8
    parents' support needs identification, 165–6
    service provider training, 166–7
  family support, 169, 170–1
  inter-agency collaboration, 169, 170
  postnatal depression screening, 64–5
  service provider training, 169, 170

Barnados Willow Project, 122
Bath and North East Somerset unitary authority, 173
  inter-agency working
    case examples, 174–7
    strategies for change, 177–9, 180
Bayley Scale of Infant Development, 53
Befriending schemes, 6
Bethlem Mother–Infant Interaction Scale (BMIS), 52
Bipolar disorder *see* Manic depressive illness
Boundaries, 87

Care in the community, 17, 64, 107, 109
  specialist services, 113–14, 137
Care Programme approach, 17
Carers (Recognition and Services) Act (1996), 110, 139
Chicago Mothers' Project, 34, 44–5, 46
Child assessment, 89–90
  case example, 90–3
Child care facilities, 25
Child protection registers, 114–15, 157, 158
Child psychiatric problems, 111
  interventions, 112
  predisposing factors, 112
Child-centred service facilities, 24–5, 106, 115
Child-rearing practices, ethnocultural aspects, 79, 80
Childhood stress see Parental mental illness, impact on children
Children Act (1989), 49, 52, 61, 69, 111, 137, 139, 157
  care/supervision orders, 74–5
Children as carers, 3, 24, 27, 75, 87, 110, 122, 163, 168
  Adventure Weekend Breaks Project, 139–40
  case example, 176
  parents' perspective, 101
  support needs, 6
Children's rights, 20, 164
Children's service plans, 119, 120, 161
Cognitive development, 53, 89
Communication
  ethnic minority groups, 116
  inter-agency working, case example, 174, 175
  protocols, 119–20, 125
Community Care Act (1990), 137, 139
Community Care Charter, 120
Community Care Plan, 120
Community resources, 8
Compulsory sterilization programmes, 29–31, 47

Confidentiality, 24, 25, 188
Conflict of interest, 1, 4, 15, 23–4, 33–4, 52, 69–72, 173, 187
  case examples, 87–9
  risk management, 71–2, 107–8
  service approaches, 70–1
Contraception, 40, 41, 44
Coping strategies, 116
  parents' perspective, 102–3
Cumulative risk, 12

Delusional systems, 2, 26, 72, 76, 77, 89
  impact on children, 91, 92, 94, 112
Depressive illness, 2, 20, 72, 73, 86, 156, 174, 186
  child abuse prediction, 115
  homicides, 112
  impact on children, 15, 20, 75, 111
  inpatient-overrepresentation of women, 17
  symptoms, 20
Development assessment, 53, 89
Disability Discrimination Act (1995), 33
Discriminatory practices, 35–7
  in child abuse prediction, 115, 116
Drug misuse, 4, 15, 20, 35
  child abuse prediction, 74, 115
  policy guidelines, 185–6

Edinburgh Postnatal Depression Scale, 65
Emotional abuse, 11, 18
Emotional deprivation, 24, 75, 86
  ethnocultural aspects, 83
Environmetal risk factors, 18–19
Epidemiology of mental illness, 17, 18
Ethnocultural aspects, 78–95, 116, 161
  case examples, 84–6, 87–9, 93–5
  child-rearing practices, 79, 80
  childrens' needs, 6
  communication, 84–5, 116
  family assessment, 79, 81–4

assessment of child, 89–93
  assessment of parent, 86–9
  family structure, 79–81, 82–3
  life cycle issues, 79–81
  parenting assessment, 50, 82
  rituals of family life, 83–4
  service organization, 93, 95
Euthanasia programmes, 31

Failure to reach competency, 18
Family assessment, 79, 81–4
  assessment of child, 89–93
  assessment of parent, 86–9
  ethnocultural case examples, 84–6,
    87–9, 90–3
  ethnocultural communication, 84–5
'FamilyBridge' multi-agency resource,
  146–7
Family functioning levels, 6–7
Family structure, 63–4, 65
  ethnocultural aspects, 79–81, 82–3
Family support, 1–9, 15–16, 34, 35, 42,
  44, 119
  anti-discrimination principles, 32–3
  Australian services, 169, 170–1
  care/service groups, 4
  case example, 121–2
  Chicago Mothers' project, 44–5, 46
  childrens' needs, 5–6
  inter-agency collaboration, 7–9,
    20–1, 121, 169
  long-term, 7, 8
  parenting clinic, 111
  pilot projects, 3–4
  resources, 8
  role of individual practitioner, 8
  service provision, 4–7, 121–3
Family therapy, 27
Family Welfare Association (FWA)
  services, 156
Fatal child abuse, 45, 46, 64, 74, 114,
  182–5, 188
  media coverage, 46–7
  risk factors, 25
  see also Homicides

Fetal alcohol syndrome, 26
Fluctuating parental responsiveness, 2

Genetic aspects, 10, 34
  bipolar disorder, 10, 19
  compulsory sterilzation programmes,
    29, 30, 31
  informed choice, 41–2
  learning disabilities, 56
  parental rights, 37–8
  schizophrenia, 10, 19, 34, 111
  stigma, 41, 42
GPs
  fund-holding problems, 119
  inter-agency communication, 188
  training, 179

Health authority purchasing
  arrangements, 119
Holistic perspective, 4, 15–16, 138,
  187, 188
Home care, 5
  domestic support for children, 6
Homicides, 1, 8, 20, 109, 112
  see also Fatal child abuse
Hospital visits, 98, 106

Icarus project, 3
Information giving, 105–6
  for children, 2, 3, 5, 6
Inter-agency service provision, 95
  Australian services, 169, 170
  barriers, 142–3, 180–1
  Bath and North East Somerset unitary
    authority, 173–81
  case responsibilities, 141–2
  fragmentation, 116–18
  collaborative protocols, 127–8,
    129–36
  communication protocols, 119–20,
    125, 126–36
  communications breakdown, 174,
    175
  family support, 7–9, 20–1, 169
  guidelines, 141, 142, 144

risk assessment checklists, 142
Lewisham experience see Lewisham service organization
referral routes, 118, 126
resources, 118–19, 142, 145
service integration, 110–13
specialisms, 113–15, 137–9, 142
supervised contact at The Meeting House, 160–1
training, 120, 142, 144, 179
Inter-generational mental illness, 8, 27, 110

Learning disabilities
  genetic aspects, 56
  parenting assessment, 55–7
    case example, 57–8
  social deprivation, 56–7
Lewisham service organization, 137–55
  adventure weekends, 139–40
  'FamilyBridge' multi-agency resource, 146–7
  joint agency work research project, 140–7
    questionnaire, 149–55
    recommendations, 143–4, 145
Lithium, 20
Local authority responsibilities, 14, 119
  joint agency work, 141–2
Long-term family support, 7, 8
Loss of custody, 32, 35, 36, 42–3, 45, 46, 99–100, 110
  case examples, 58, 61, 174
  impact on parents, 113
  parental fears, 36, 110, 116, 166, 168
  risk of violence, 74–5
Loss of parenting role, 97–100
Low birthweight, 11

Manic depressive illness, 3, 19–20, 29, 31, 96, 110, 147, 164
  case example, 176
    impact on children, 147–9
  genetic aspects, 10, 19, 41
  relapse following childbirth, 19

symptoms, 19–20
Marce Society, 64, 68
Material needs, 103
Media coverage, 46–7, 107, 109.
Medication
  compliance, 60, 61, 76
  side effects, 2, 27, 39, 98
Meeting Place, The (Thomas Coram Foundation contact centre), 157–62
  case example, 158–9
  supervision of contact, 158, 159
    outcomes, 159–60
Mental Health Act (1983), 69, 72
Mental Health Services Charter, 120
Mental illness
  acute, 72, 75–6
  case studies, 73–4
  chronic persistent illness, 73, 75
  definitions, 72–4
  recurrent symptoms, 73
  risk of violence, 74, 75–6
  social isolation, 75
  threat-control-override (TCO) symptoms, 74
MIND 'Breakthrough' campaign, 156
Mother and Baby Units, 49, 52, 53, 64, 106, 123
Motor development assessment, 53

Neglect, 79
  see also Emotional deprivation
Neurotic disorders
  impact on children, 26
  inpatient-overrepresentation of women, 17
New Parent Infant Network (NEWPIN), 156
NSPCC family support project, 157

Obessional/compulsive disorders
  case study, 21–2
  impact on children, 26

Parent support groups, 5
Parental mental illness, 34–5

discriminatory practices, 35–7
impact on children, 1–4, 26, 47,
    52–3, 75, 78, 110, 111, 161, 165
  assessment, 89, 90
  attachment relationships disruption,
    54–5
  Australian Research Project,
    167–8
  chronic persistent versus discrete
    episodes, 2
  denial, 26
  schizophrenia, 59
  labelling effects, 115
  Lewisham Social Services joint
    agency work research project,
    140–7
  overrepresentation of women, 17, 18
  prevalence, 18
  risk to children, 1, 2, 4, 18
  user's perspective, 96–108
    becoming a parent, 100–1
    coping strategies, 102–3
    information giving, 105–6
    loss of parenting role, 97–100
    professional responses, 103–5
    role reversal, 101–2
Parental reactive stress, 15
Parental responsibilities, 14–15
  ethnocultural aspects, 80
Parental rights, 14, 164
  genetic aspects, 37–8
  right to have children, 28–48, 55
    anti-discrimination principles,
      32–4
    discriminatory practices/attitudes,
      35–7, 44
    informed choice, 40–2, 44
  termination, 35–6, 47
Parenting assessment, 49–62
  comprehensive approach, 51–2
  infants, 53–5
  learning disabilities, 55–7
    case example, 57–8
  problems, 50–1, 62
  schizophrenia, 59–60

  case example, 60–2
Parenting capability, 24–5
  ethnocultural aspects, 82
  family support approach, 4–5
  parental rights issues, 28, 31–2
  social workers' focus, 104
  sociocultural aspects, 65
Parenting clinic support, 111
Pathology focus of social workers,
  103–4
Peer support groups, 171
Perinatal mental disorders, 3, 63–8
  predisposing factors, 66
  prevention, 66–8
Perinatal support services, 3
Personality disorder, 2, 36
  case study, 22
  homicides, 112
  inpatient-overrepresentation of
    women, 17
  risk to children, 18, 115
Phobic disorders, 26, 27
Physical child abuse, 11, 79
  parental stress association, 111
  see also Fatal child abuse
Post-partum psychoses, 79
Post-traumatic stress disorders, 12, 72,
  73
Postnatal depression, 3, 96, 100, 156
  case example, 176
  family support, 122–3
  prevention, 66–8
  see also Perinatal mental disorders
Pregnancy, ethnocultural aspects, 79, 80
Prematurity, 11
Professional network, 78–9
Professionals' responsibilites, 14–15
Psychiatric ward facilities, 42
Psychotic illness, 75
  family disruption, 167
  impact on children, 26, 27
  inpatient-overrepresentation of
    women, 17
  perinatal disorders, 3
  suicide risk, 73

Rape, 39–40, 109
Referral routes, 118, 126
Rehabilitation, 36–7, 42, 48, 115
Residential family assessment centres, 35
Resilience in children, 11, 165
Respite care, 5, 33
 Adventure Weekend Breaks Project, 139–40
Right to have children *see* Parental rights
Right to Life movement, 38
Risk to children, 10–16
 assessment, 45, 49–62, 72–7, 115–16, 183, 184, 187–8
  inter-agency communication, 184, 188
  see also Parenting assessment
 conflict of interest, 71–2, 107–8
 environmental factors, 12–13
 expectations of public, 71
 management, 71
  safe management structures, 71–2
 mental illness association, 74
 nature of harm, 11–12
 risk perception, 70
 unacceptable risk, 13, 74–7

Salford Community Health Trust, 122
Schizophrenia, 19, 29, 30, 31, 34, 96, 164
 ability to care for children, 19, 45, 47, 59, 60, 116, 168
 case examples, 21, 60–2, 76, 85–6, 87–8, 90–5, 163, 183–5
 co-morbidity, 14
 communication, 85–6
 family support, 123
 genetic aspects, 10, 19, 34, 41, 42, 111
 impact on children, 27, 111, 122, 163
 parenting assessment, 59–62
 symptoms, 19
School failure, 90
Second marriages, 100–1

Self-harm, 2
 case studies, 21, 22
Service protocols, 8
Service provision, 109–36, 182–8
 child-centred facilities, 106
 discriminatory practices, 115, 116
 family support, 121–3
 Health Advisory Service model, 119, 124
 integration of services, 110–13
  specialisms, 113–15, 137
 joint working *see* Inter-agency service provision
 organizational arrangements, 119–21
 parents' perspective, 103–5
  affirmation of strengths, 104
  child-centred focus, 105
  negative parenting capacity assessment, 104
  pathology focus, 103–4
 risk assessment, 115–16
Sexual abuse, 11
 subsequent psychiatric disorders, 112, 184, 185
Sexual activity, 38–9
Sexual assault, 39–40
Sexual orientation, discriminatory practices, 116
Single parenting, 66, 98, 102
Sleep clinic, 123
Social disadvantage, 13–14, 24, 29, 34, 35, 42, 137, 165
 benefit policies, 37
 learning disabilities, 56–7
Social isolation, 75
Social workers' responsibilities, 105
Specialization, 113–15, 137–9, 142, 175
 barriers to communication, 175
 communication protocols, 119–20, 125
Step-parenting, 101
Stigma-associated stresses, 6, 27, 89, 99
Suicide, 73, 109, 185

Supervised contact, 159, 160
Supervision registers, 114–15

Targetting support, 6
Temperament, 10, 11, 165
Thomas Coram Foundation contact
  centre (The Meeting Place), 157–62
Threat-control-override (TCO)
  symptoms, 74, 76, 77
Threshold Mothers' Project, 33
Timescales, 15, 90

Training, 120, 123, 184, 186
  Australian services, 169, 170
  inter-agency work, 142, 144, 179
Triangulation method, 140

Voluntary sector projects, 156–62

Wallington Resource Centre, 122
Women's psychiatric illness, 17
Woodley Enquiry Report, 2, 109, 123
Workload, 186